Transitions

Writings from the
University of New Hampshire
Composition Program

University of New Hampshire

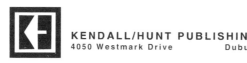

KENDALL/HUNT PUBLISHING COMPANY
4050 Westmark Drive   Dubuque, Iowa 52004

Contents

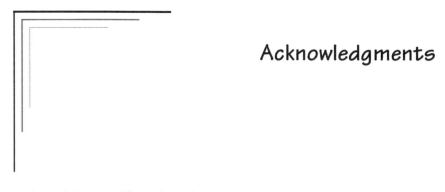

Acknowledgments

Transitions would not have been possible without the help of the following people: Abby Knoblauch, for her tireless work on the selection committee and tackling too many administrative details to mention here; Dr. Jessica Enoch, for her work on the selection committee; Dr. John Ernest, for his new vision of *Transitions*; Dr. Paul Matsuda, for helping with the final details; and Joe Sabella, at Kendall/Hunt for all of his enthusiasm and support.

A Message from the Director of Undergraduate Composition

Welcome to the University of New Hampshire and to English 401, First-Year Writing. As you probably know, English 401 is the only course virtually all UNH students take during their first year. It is also the first of a series of writing intensive courses. As such, it is uniquely situated to facilitate the development of college-level literacy skills that will serve you as you encounter various writing situations throughout your college career and beyond.

The primary mission of English 401 is to help you develop the ability to use writing effectively in personal, academic and professional contexts. You will practice various strategies that are important in college-level writing, such as: understanding the rhetorical situation, including the task, purpose, audience, and genre; identifying and developing topics; developing and organizing ideas; evaluating, incorporating and citing sources; drafting and revising; giving and receiving feedback; editing and proofreading; and using styles that are appropriate for the rhetorical situation. To accomplish the course objectives, your instructor will use a combination of various modes of instruction—such as lectures, discussion, small-group workshops, in- and out-of-class writing, and individual and group conferences.

In this course, you can expect to encounter four types of writing: personal writing, analytic writing, research writing, and persuasive writing.

- Personal writing will help you reflect on and explore your own experience and knowledge, and in the process, generate new insights that can be shared with an audience.

- Analytic writing will provide tools for critically examining various artifacts and practices, and for communicating your observations and interpretations to an audience.

- Research writing will emphasize the importance of formulating genuine and generative research questions, of collecting and organizing supporting and counter evidence, and of developing and presenting informed arguments in a professional voice appropriate for an academic audience.

• Persuasive writing will help you engage in the discussion of various issues effectively by providing tools for considering different perspectives and for presenting your argument not only by constructing logical arguments but also by establishing your credibility and by addressing the reader's feelings.

These types of writing differ in emphases but are not mutually exclusive—they overlap and work together in various writing situations. For this reason, your instructor will assign these types of writing in a combination of a range of real-world writing genres, some of which are represented in the volume you are holding in your hands.

In addition, English 401 provides opportunities to learn how to use tools and resources that are essential to your success as a college-level writer, such as library resources, writing handbooks, computer resources, and the writing center.

Your college-level literacy development will not stop at the end of this course because every writing situation is unique and presents you with a new set of challenges, as some of the examples in this book will attest. I hope what you learn in English 401 will help you as you respond to those challenges and continue to grow as a writer.

Paul Kei Matsuda, Ph.D.
Director of Undergraduate Composition

Section 1

Writings from the
University of New Hampshire
Composition Program

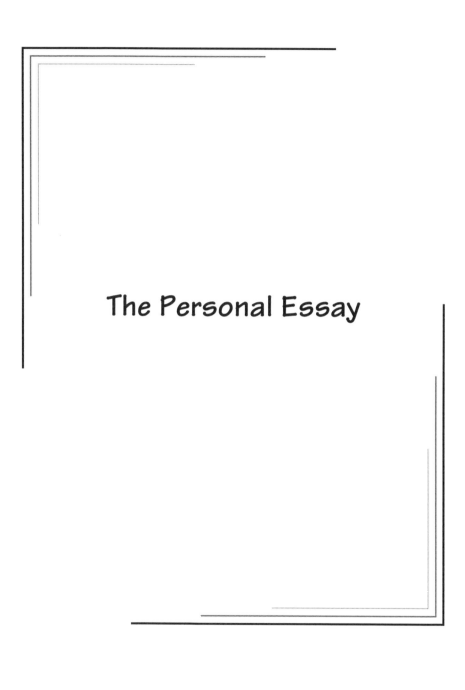

The Personal Essay

Cloaked

1

Elizabeth A. Joseph

Outside of Dad's workroom, the four of us converged—whispering quietly. Suggestions which border-lined demands to open the door carried throughout, bouncing off the basement's brick walls.

he's gotta be in there

open the door

Excuses followed quickly.

I can't reach the latch

you're the oldest

yeah well, you're always saying you're not afraid of anything…prove it

are you sure you checked all the closets?

I had checked the closets four thousand times. I had checked in-between every shirt hanging therein. I had memorized the order in which they fell. The closets were checked—Dad wasn't there.

Tonight started like all the other nights: stupid kitchen duty and all its drying of plates was over; school uniforms were ready; lunch-bags were labeled and juice boxes appropriately placed inside; mix-matching pajamas from the PJ basket were on; homework had been completed hours before; syllable-by-syllable words floated in our heads for our ritual and respective spelling tests. Hide-n-go-seek-in-the-house emerged as the game of choice after a week where too many vases had been broken, too many picture frames had fallen from the walls, too many windows held a baseball sized stencil, and too many *Nerf* or Nothin' footballs had flown over the neighbor's fence. The only requisite was that it was nighttime and our only preference was that all the lights be turned off anyway. The first was satisfied always. The latter, almost never.

We always hid first, then Dad. Most nights, when it was our turn to find, we split up to search and boasted with a loud *I found him*! when we did. Generally we hid three times and Dad three times before bed. Our neighbors, Al and Eleanor, easily followed the game as they sat on their porch eating dinner (yeah, we went to bed *that* early).

That night we had only hidden once. Each room had been double-tri-pled-quadrupled checked. We each had gone our own ways to claim vic-tory and all returned to the living room puzzled and apprehensive—*did you find him? No one found him yet?* We moved to the omniscient source of whom we were certain could be bribed with hugs (or if that failed, prom-ises to clean our rooms).

Mom, where is he? Come on . . . where?

I don't know.

We won't tell, promise.

Pleaaase . . . we looked everywhere.

She really didn't know. Or so she still claims.

Try checking the rooms again?

What else was there to do? We left Mom sitting on the couch to her sewing box and ripped school uniforms, and for the first time in the histo-ry of our game, we checked the rooms together. Four small wanderers: two boys, two girls, in that age order, with missing teeth and scraped knees. And one mystery father who had the power to disappear—had Bil-bo's One Ring in his possession and was using it in a game of hide-n-go-seek-in-the-house. We discovered he had the Ring when he reappeared hours later to four bemused kids taking council on the living room car-pet—to a white faced Rebekah, Mark fidgeting with the rug fringe, An-thony's eyes darting around waiting for Dad to pop out at us, and me sitting Indian-style on the fresh apple juice stain Mom hadn't noticed yet. He came up the cellar stairs the same Dad as before he disappeared, Old

Spice, running sneakers, full beard, but grinning like he was Bilbo himself returning triumphant to the Shire. Loud shrieks and a wild race ensued.

Where were you?!

You didn't see me?

Dad, where were you hiding?

I wasn't…I was following you guys around.

What?

I used the Ring, he told us. We tried to mouth, you have *the* Ring? but our jaws only dropped as we looked up, wide-eyed, at our jubilant father.

A decade later at Thanksgiving we would find out he was in the workroom the whole time. He heard us whispering outside, heard our footsteps run from the shadows. He watched from behind the workroom door as we slowly pushed it open and stared in. He swears he made eye-contact with one of us. We all sat at the Thanksgiving table listening to the truth of our suspicions, believing less than completely his claim. Memory, while lenient with persuasion and over time, is less than willing to change immediately. Over the years we had come to terms that he had probably been in the workroom and we too wild in our imaginations as kids to stay and look fully. Maybe it's that memory works hand in hand with imagination—both feeding off the other, catalyst or host. My past is host to me. I host to my memory. Changes to that memory are unwelcome, at best. Unless I let them in—or more honestly, truth forces entrance. Looking right through it all: my father was invisible to us then, and remains a matter of perception in my memory now. Two endings to this story present themselves, and for all logical reasons, I should tell the actual version. Late in my teenage years, after understanding the reality, I tell the preferred, authentic ending—as it was then: perplexed kids, a dexterous father, a powerful ring.

No, you were in the workroom . . . weren't you?

You said you looked there, did you see me?

We did look there. Anthony decided it would be best if we opened the door together. He was the oldest and tallest so he would lift the latch;

Mark was next in age so he would push the blue paint-chipped door open slowly; all four of us would look. Three-fourth's open—empty: a 5x10 room, smelling of paint, metal, old paper. Dimly lit with a pull-string bulb. Perfect for a mildew science experiment: dry in the winter, damp in the summer. Hammers, nails, scary water-heater, broken exercise bike, fragmented wood, spray-paint, tool-box, countless tools, light bulbs, phone cords, paint, tarp, folding chairs, outdated board games, shelves of things that can only be described as "things," light switch covers, tiles, doorknobs, tea-kettle, shoelaces, crates, Styrofoam, cardboard, super-glue, scrap-box, Chimney Sweeping Logs, frayed rugs, drill-bits, chewed pencils, sawdust, a Noah's ark pillow case fronting as a curtain, tire pump, deflated basketballs, old books, dust-mask, AM/FM radio, used micro-wave, rubber gloves. We thought we saw it all. Dad stuff. No Dad.

Dad, we did look there...

He shrugged as he sat down on the couch and folded the newspaper to the crossword puzzle and probably grinned or winked at Mom beside him. His only reply for us was bed time. I can only imagine how badly he wanted to tell us—at that moment and the years thereafter. In a way, he preserved our imaginations—countless times we had discussed possibilities of where he hid. And every time, our only answer was that he had the greatest of the Rings of Power. Long before any of us had heard of J.R.R. Tolkien's trilogy in which the Ring is established as a ring of doom (and with which we would live and love years later) we were mesmerized with its prequel of sorts, *The Hobbit*. Bilbo and his journey there and back again: through Middle Earth to the Lonely Mountain and back to the Shire and sometime during his journey he met my father and passed the Ring of power on. This Ring which turns its wearer invisible. We were dumbfounded (had we really never noticed his wedding ring before?)— the Ring. One simple gold band to solve our mystery—a father's tale.

After that game, and our discovery, we decided it was only fair that the Ring not be used when we played hide-n-go-seek-in-the-house. We also suggested that the workroom be off limits during game-time, hardly a place for kids to be wandering in, nails and all that. (Though, all four of us would later admit that room was a childhood fear.) Both requests were agreed to and we never had too much trouble finding Dad again. Except in our memories. There, he stands both in the workroom and cloaked be-side our wandering silhouettes about, over, and through the house—all in an adventure of invisible proportions.

2

Spies

Nathaniel Lord

We were never the type of people to be proud of our heritage. That's not to say we were ashamed, we just didn't care. We didn't feel the need to attend Scottish or French festivals put on at the The Elks or The Loyal Order of the Moose. My Memere can date her ancestry to her parents whereas my Grammy can date the family back further but just chooses not to talk about it. I can't think of one time of hearing about my ancestors in Europe as if they were exiled and were not to be discussed. The only point discussed is that I'm a direct descendent of Nathan Hale, but nobody in the family knows anything about him other than that he's in the *Encyclopedia Britannica* (although no family members have bothered to read the small article). In American History in high school we went over the Revolution and for obvious reasons Nathan came up. I raised my hand. "What did he do? I mean, like, in the revolution—what did he *do*?"

"He was a soldier for the Americans," said Mr. Hawley.

"I think he said 'don't fire until you see the whites of their eyes' or something," contributed a student.

"Yeah, that sounds right," said the teacher, and we moved on.

How vague and sad. How sad that my ancestor is summed up in two sentences. They were both wrong by the way. He was not a soldier, he was a spy and he said before his execution, "I only regret that I have but one life to lose for my country." What a badass. To basically spit in the face of your enemy before they kill you, to be hung, to die, and now to be almost forgotten, as a spy would want it.

At three o'clock in some autumn month in seventh grade, I got off the bus at my Memere's. Mom stood there alone, her hand tied behind her back by her fingers. Her eyes were puffy and her short merlot hair seemed to bother her as I got off the bus—it was an excuse not to look directly at me. Her mouth opened, not round but as a bar, trying to not cry but she wants to. Fuck, not my sisters. Somebody's dead. Not my sisters. Anybody but Helen or Claire. Fuck. Shit. I hug Mom and she forces an exhale.

My Grandpa had died. He was round with white hair and a white, un-kempt beard—the kind stained light brown around the mouth as if he ate coffee ice cream with every meal. Grandpa lived in Florida with Pricilla. I never knew what she was. After the wake my mom introduced Pricilla to a distant relative, the type that drive from an unknown state and view a wake as an excuse for a long weekend.

"Carol, this is Pricilla, my Dad's gir-"

"I was his friend," she cut my mom off politely. She introduced herself as his friend to everyone. But they lived together. I slept over at *their* house. Why didn't she say she was his girlfriend? Who is she? They slept in the same bedroom, that I'm sure of, but in separate twin beds like in *I Love Lucy*. Was he just a good friend? Or maybe Pricilla was a secret rela-tive? Or was he gay? Maybe they broke up right before his death. Or were they just private with those matters?

We had a connection, or at least he wanted to have one with me. He was one of the only relatives I had that would not talk to me about how tall I was. When I reached a certain age, I believe eleven (or was it twelve? It doesn't matter.) Grandpa took me up north, that is to say to the north-ern part of New Hampshire, first with my Mom's family, then alone. He showed me the North, his St. Kitts, but never anything truly personal about himself. He would tell incomplete stories, like how an old lady by where he lived made soap out of bull's fat, or about the time he was drunk and a friend paid him in a wad of twenties to take him to California that night to see the Pacific. He never gave all the facts, just enough for the story to make sense, unless he talked about his brother.

The few times he talked about my great-uncle (I don't know his name, I don't think he told me), Grandpa would start out and end by shaking his head and saying that he was brilliant, so bright. Grandpa would tell me that his brother at the age of five knew how to operate a tractor by himself on their family's farm. His brother was very "good with math and things like that," which would be followed with the shake of his head while look-ing down. "Brilliant, so bright. It's such a shame he had to be taken away, but I guess with a mind like his there's you know, good and bad that comes with it. It's such a damn shame he had to be taken away. He was brilliant." And then the subject was changed like the flipping of a chan-nel.

The North Country is far different from southern New Hampshire. It's kind of like Alaska without the cold and polar bears. It's a place of single trailer parks placed on dirt roads with scraps of junk in the front yard. But why would they care to clean it up? There's no keeping up with the Jone-ses when there are no Joneses. It is a place where the national border of

Canada and the U.S. doesn't seem to matter. The people that live here don't care about such trivial concerns.

Our transportation to the North Country was his old car from the fifties. It was baby blue and in poor condition. It looked . . . beautiful. Like when you see an old man or woman and they show you a picture of themselves in their mid-twenties and you no longer see the person as old but as a beautiful person; you see through their wrinkles. The car had no seat belts, only two doors, and smelled of sweat and dust. The back of the Cadillac was filled with items he collected over the past year, all of which blocked the rear window.

His friends in the North Country were much younger than Grandpa, most in their mid-thirties. There was a man with only three fingers on one of his hands, a woman who would yell a lot like she was always drunk and various other characters. I have no idea how he met these people. He at no time in his life lived in the North Country, but he acted like he had known these people for quite a long time. How he had time to travel on a regular basis more than three hours, meet people in a town that is as random as any on the map, and become friends with them I don't know.

Grandpa would show up at our house with steamers and raw oysters every few weekends. Whenever he ate an oyster he would always check for pearls. He taught me how to eat a steamer every time he came over, as if I forgot each time. First you open the shell and pull out the steamer. There could be some meat still left in the shell, don't forget about that; don't waste it. Pull off the skin from the neck—you don't want to eat that. First dip the stomach of the steamer in the clam water, then in butter, then eat it. The neck is tough, so be careful not to choke; don't throw away the neck, it's good but it's tough.

At the end of the wake me, Mom, Andria my sister, Pricilla, and my aunt had to stand by the casket so people could pay their respects to us as they said goodbye to Grandpa. I didn't want to see them; I didn't want to be there so I squeezed my mom's hand and cried. My mouth was dry and filled with sticky spit. I don't want to be here. Mom thanked people as they passed by and I left the line. In the parlor, I guess you would call it, of the funeral home, about ten minutes later Andria joined me.

"I don't want to be here," I said.

"I know," she said and hugged me in the way that older sisters can and squeezed me hard.

The last time I saw Grandpa was when I was over at his house for some reason. He wanted to take me on a road trip in an RV he was thinking of buying. The kitchen had only one dim light over the table in the center of the room. I was eating a piece of chicken pizza left over from the day before that was cold. Grandpa was already excited about the trip months in the future and was writing down a list of what we were going to need: spam, bread, milk, butter, eggs. He was ready to go mentally and I'm certain if we had supplies and RV, he would want to leave that night. He died later that week. The doctor said it was a heart problem, but I'm not sure what it was exactly. He was alone working on a project and fell over. He was found the next morning.

The priest spoke, saying that he didn't know Grandpa personally, but he was a good man. Most everybody nodded their heads silently. "He was a good man"—a summary of over sixty years of existence.

I walked to the casket and looked at Grandpa not in a suit, but a tee-shirt and jeans. I put my head over my mouth to stop a laugh that never came. Who is he? No doubt he insisted on being buried this way. I put my hands behind my back and squeezed them. I took my mom and we exited the church to the graveyard, descendants of a spy burying one of their own.

Between Two Worlds

3

Preethi Nath

My mind wanders on a journey through the blur of this afternoon. I am standing alongside my mother in the kitchen preparing curry for the first time. Mother's guarding, discerning artist's eyes focus on the changing shades, and I observe how she carefully sifts through the portions with her hands. Yet although I watch her, I do not imitate her. I hold the chicken tightly and bathe it in the curry; rolling until I find my own rhythm. My curry making surprises my parents, since they see me as the daughter who has lost her culture.

But today, as I coat the chicken with curry, my hands are drawn out as if to extend across the ocean that separates my parents from me. While my parents' physical presence lays in America, their hearts lie attached to India. They are still fixated in the ways of the Old Country and in their minds I have become too Westernized—only capable of mumbling awkward sentences in Hindi and unknowing of the significance of the ancient texts of the Vedas and Upanishads. They would like me to be more Indian but they do not know what it is like to grow up in two different cultures and not know where to belong.

But my parents have sacrificed much for me that makes this cultural rift between us insignificant. I want to make up for the silent dinners and the stereotypes we cast on each other and look into the eyes of my parents who are silently questioning my faith and culture and tell them that I understand. I have not experienced their life under the hot Indian sun, and my father's stories of growing up on a farm in a small Indian village and walking to school five miles everyday in the blazing sun seems so distant. To me, they are only stories of an old life, relics of a fading past. But I need to know them, to understand them beyond words. I have to feel the emotions, to engross myself in identity and search for meaning.

My parents came to America absorbed in their past lives, the precious pieces of their existence carted off into a few economy-sized suitcases as they marched toward an uncertain future. Clutching onto their past with a sack of silk, gold, and spices, they moved forward. Yet everything to that point had become meaningless. They began to build new lives—their own identities in a world of strange faces. And it was hard. Every day was spent searching for a sort of security that they couldn't find, and every night was wasted wondering when they could stop looking. My father came to America upon graduating from medical school and completed his board exams in search of a residency. While my father applied for residencies, my mother scrambled in search of jobs to cover the expenses of their small, worn-down apartment on the edges of the rough section of Brooklyn. Their lives were full of far-off dreams that called to them. Yet everything kept moving, with or without them, for better or for worse.

In those years, my parents overcame tremendous adversity. The first time they stepped off the platform, they were introduced to the word "Paki," by an angry man aboard the train. "Paki" was a derogatory term for people of Pakistani and Indian descent. Thus, in this new land, they had to fight not only to live but against the racism that discretely thrived under the pockets of civil society. Yet despite the obstacles in their way, they worked hard and persevered. They were the epitome of the American Dream. Knowing that academics were the ticket to economic stability and success, my parents placed a high value on educational achievements and set high academic standards for me. They firmly believed that with hard work and perseverance I could be anything and wanted me to take full advantage of every opportunity that I had.

However, growing up I sometimes felt like I couldn't measure up to their standards. So, if I got a poor grade on a test or paper, I would hide it in my room, afraid that if they knew about it they would love me less for my imperfections. I yearned for my parents' love and affection and I thought that by trying to project an image of the perfect daughter they would be happy and take pride in me. So an enormous conflict for me was trying to understand my parents' thinking, why they valued academics to such a high standard, and to realize that they really wanted what was best for me but just didn't know how to express that.

Over twenty years have passed since they left India. And in those years, I have grown up in a world completely different from my parents. As a second-generation American, I struggled with the difficulty of choosing between the Indian values that I was raised with and the need to assimilate to American culture. Desperate for mainstream acceptance, but at the same time wanting to preserve my culture, I resorted to a double life. Like a chameleon changing color, I changed my roles. With my friends I was American, and with my parents I was Indian. I kept family and social life separate, yet by doing so I felt a false sense of fulfilling my responsibilities.

The opposing values and beliefs of two worlds continually collided and I felt caught in an identity tug-of-war. My family ties weakened in my attempts to distance myself from my Indian identity. All I had wanted was acceptance, a misguided notion of the embodiment of American moral values.

And then this past summer I visited India. The last time I had visited India I was only twelve and too young to understand the beautiful complexity of India and its people. Looking back, it's as if I lived several lives in the span of four months. I've enjoyed mountains, the seas, the heat and humidity of Calcutta; the chill and mist of Darjeeling, yet finding warmth there, too; the many cultures and languages, the clip-pity-clop of the beat along various tracks, the deep orange-blotted sunsets and firing-squad lightening storms; the broken streets; the kind eyes of strangers who were friends in disguise; the various horns coming to wake me even when I thought I was awake; the sights of rickshaw drivers giving money to child beggars—and feeling humbled by it. I'll remember the hands of those young and old, all in motion. India is motion standing still. Leafing through my journal, I read a sentence I wrote on my first day in India: "Nothing has happened . . . yet so much has happened." In India, I discovered my roots—that being Indian was such a large part of my identity that I would be lost by renouncing it. Even more importantly, I realized that true acceptance could only be gained by acceptance of self and that by distancing myself from my heritage, I was denying a large part of who I was.

And I start to understand. I take out the curry from the oven and set it aside on the table, breathing in the strong aroma. The food is a part of me. Every time I sense the smell of curry, I am reminded of who I am, of those much anticipated birthday parties as a child and of the joy I felt as I helped my mother cook. Sitting at the kitchen table, my five-year-old fingers bathed in curry, my mother and I would have heart-to-heart discussions of the most trivial things, whose topics I no longer remember, but of which I never tired. My parents' stories are a part of who I am, and who I will become. Their legacy is the only possession worth keeping, for once forgotten it will never come back. We came here not to escape the memories, but to hold onto them; to fulfill a life that no one in our family has never known and I hope to preserve them.

4

Grey Skies

Marisha Florissant

I have never been to England, but today I could imagine what it might look like on a dreary December morning. It's one of those days when the grey skies sink down into the forests and towns, concealing sharp lines and color. I'm on my way to Keene in the backseat of a late 90s Ford Escort. My boyfriend, Nathan, sits shot-gun as his older brother, Zak, drives us out of town. I settle in behind Nathan and try to start a conversation with his brother's girlfriend who was bundled up in wool and seated to my right. Unfortunately, after exchanging greetings and inquiring about her flight in from the city, the conversation fizzles from lack of anything in common.

I look out the window at the land that time forgot. All small towns look similar up here; they lack developed business areas and busy intersections. Many small New Hampshire towns are filled with old farm houses, fields, and the occasional country-themed mansion of a wealthy family looking to escape the city. Some towns are noticeably poorer and display old broken down pick-up trucks; trailers parked next to small decaying houses look metallic and cold. Overall the scenery is mostly the same and has remained this way my whole life. By the time we've reached Keene, the fog had settled in and turned into a mist, the kind of mist that never really turns into a rain but will soak anything left outside for too long. We turn into a short gravel driveway that separates a large open yard from an old townhouse; my hands shake with apprehension.

A few months ago Nathan was diagnosed with a very rare and serious form of cancer. The news might as well have thrown me down an elevator shaft. In the aftermath of the diagnosis, Nathan and I hold hands a lot. There are days when I feel as though I might slide off the edge of the earth if he wasn't there for me to hold on to. People take for granted the satisfaction of holding hands. To witness a couple's intertwined fingers is routine and is easily forgotten. My memory struggles to save every moment we share.

Through a string of unfortunate events, I am in town for the holidays, and am able to stay with him during winter break; this includes celebrating Christmas with his family. It's New Year's Eve Day, and everyone is gathering in Keene to celebrate a belated Christmas. I follow Nathan into a large white townhouse, complete with forest green porch, chipped paint, and weather worn shed. Inside, I am introduced to his grandmother whom I have met before. She looks up at me with a smile and wraps her frail arms around my back. I feel like I have just had a growth spurt leaving me tall, lanky, and awkward. The smell of roasting meat and pine engulfs me. I follow Nathan, as he walks toward the sound of jumbled conversations and laughter. All of his family is gathered into a corner room fitted with a Christmas tree that takes up an entire entrance. I gladly take a seat next to Mollie, Nathan's older sister, and seek refuge in a friendlier girl than the one I rode down with.

While Nathan's mom gets ready to hand out the presents his dad opens a bottle of champagne. They don't cry around us; it would be like seeing a teacher outside of school, uncomfortable and out of place. I wonder if they wait until they go upstairs for the night, when they can be alone. Darkness can weaken the strong; fear can creep in and agitate the pain. Mollie has seen me at my weakest moment. She came in one night, curious of what Nathan and I had planned to do later that evening. Nathan was asleep. Immediately she noticed my tear-streaked cheeks lit up in the dark by the TV. Regardless of how hard I tried to hold it together, I couldn't answer her. She cleared the hair from my face.

"Are you okay, hun?" she whispered. I choked back the growing lump in my throat.

"Sometimes it's hard . . ." was all I could get out before the lump forced water from my eyes and abruptly ended my ability to speak. Her arms came around my shoulders, her head rested next to mine; she had also lost the fight against the lump in her throat.

Nathan's dad hands Mollie a bottle of champagne. Despite her tendency to leave her problems out of any conversations we've had, Mollie had her reasons, as did I, to keep the bottle close. Nathan's mom overpronounces my name in excitement as I am handed an unexpected gift. I can't stop smiling, as I rip into the little bag. In a furry of crinkling wrapping paper and thrashing trash bags, I focus on the bubbles tickling my nose. Nathan reaches for a present and winces in pain. He's like an innocent man standing on trial, waiting for the verdict.

Later his mom announces the end of the presents and we head into the dining room for the largest family dinner I have even attended. When we've had our fill of Christmas dinner, Nathan, Zak, his girlfriend, Mollie and I take a short drive to his grandparent's house just outside of town. This house had been deemed "The Farm House," and that is exactly what it is: red chipped paint, creaky stairs, and iron latches. There were a few sparse old pine trees near the house, but past the driveway is a field covered in matted dry grasses that tumbled down into a valley hidden by think fog. Nathan and Zak give the city girl a tour of the rustic house, while Mollie and I choose to rest up before going back into town. On an old, soft bedspread, I wonder how it feels to be married for over fifty years. My eyes follow the curves of faded vines and flowers that cover the walls, fifty years felt like an eternity. His grandparents are getting very old. I wonder if they are afraid of losing each other.

Zak told me he knew a guy who left his girlfriend after she was diagnosed with cervical cancer. He had been a friend of his during college; the past tense of friendship was strongly emphasized. Nathan's family members had each privately pulled me aside to talk. The message was always the same.

"Thank you," they would say. *Thank you?* I didn't do anything. There is nothing I can do.

We get back just in time for dessert, but I stay outside on the porch and sit down on a wicker loveseat. Considering how overcast it is, it seems unusually warm for the end of December . . . or maybe it's the champagne. Ignoring the clouds, Nathan and his brother play frisbee golf on the wet lawn, the rules of which I still don't understand, but it looks like something they started a long time ago. The mist has been replaced by a cool wind that blows through my fleece sweater every now and again. The girl I rode down with comes outside and sits down near me . . . still as quiet as before. I try to start a conversation, but give up quickly, choosing instead to quiet my own racing mind. I feel like I am at a track meet running a race. Quitting is not an option. All I can do is keep myself moving until I reach the end, no matter how painful. Luckily, the thing I always liked about track was that there was a winner at the end of every race.

I decide not to worry about the quiet girl on the porch with me. If she wanted to talk, she would. The world I see in front of me seems to be in slow motion. It looks plain and common; another rainy New England Christmas in a small town. I could see the property borders marked by an old log fence and across the yard another weathered house looms out of the fog. It has huge bare lilac bushes, almost like trees, that create a latticed wall between us. Sporadically, a car or truck slowly drives down the wet street lined with old maple trees, but other than that there is no one around. I feel that if I try hard enough, I could stay in this moment with the wind, the grey skies, and the smell of a woodstove . . . forever.

• • •

Rough Draft

I have never been to England, but I can imagine what it might look like on a dreary December morning. It was one of those days when the grey skies sink down into the forests and towns, concealing sharp lines of color. I was on my way to Keene in the backseat of an old Ford Escort. The driver was my boyfriend's older brother, Zak, who graduated from George Washington University a few years ago and has lived in D.C. ever since. He and his girlfriend had flown up to New Hampshire for the holidays and I was looking forward to talking to her about living in the city. However, after a few minutes into the drive it became painfully obvious that she felt out of place, emphasizing her quiet yet slightly aristocratic presence. She sat next to me looking out her window onto a land time forgot. All small towns have a similar look up here. They lack developed business areas and busy intersections. Many towns my size are filled with old farm houses, fields, and newer, larger houses that are set back into the forests owned by wealthy families looking to live in the country. Some towns are prominently poorer and display old broken down pick-up trucks parked next to small plan houses in need of a paint job, but overall it looks mostly the same. The fog that has settled in has turned into a mist, the kid of mist that never really turns into rain but will soak anything left outside for too long.

My boyfriend, Nathan, occupies the seat in front of me and carries on a slightly hushed conversation with his brother that is made inaudible by the music on the radio. I feel the need to be acknowledged, most likely a side effect of being an only child, so I start to massage the back of his neck and place my left hand on his shoulder. Almost as if he read my mind his hand comes up to cover mine and gives it a little squeeze. I think people take for granted the satisfaction of holding hands. For the past month now I have been more aware and grateful for the little things I enjoy.

The ride down to Keene is long and boring. Trees make up the majority of what is flying by only to be broken up by the occasional town and white steeple church. The closer we get to Keene the more often we have to change the radio station to prevent static. Despite all of this I am grateful for this trip. Three weeks ago my boyfriend was diagnosed with a very rare and serious form of cancer. The news might as well have thrown me down an elevator shaft. I swear, the floor dropped out from under me.

Since then I find that Nathan and I hold hands as often as possible. There are days when I feel as though I might slide off the edge of the earth if he wasn't there for me to hold on to. Through a convenient string of unfortunate events I was able to stay with him during winter break and that included celebrating Christmas with his family. One New Year's Eve everyone went down to Keene to celebrate a belated Christmas and to have Christmas dinner.

I usually spend Christmas with my mom and a few aunts or on rare occasions I fly out to Colorado and spend it with my father's side of the family. This trip was special to me not only because of the people I got to spend it with but also the whole experience was something I rarely got to take part in. When we finally got there we pulled up to a large white farm house, complete with weather worn shed and chipped paint. Inside I met aunts, uncles, and Nathan's grandparents and the small of dinner and pine lingered through out the rooms. We all gathered into the rooms with the Christmas tree. Everyone found a seat even if they had to pull chairs out of other rooms. I gladly took a seat next to Nathan's sister, Mollie, who is currently a junior at Stonehill College and took refuge in a friendlier girl than the one I rode down with.

While Nathan's mom handed out presents his dad opened a bottle of champagne. Due to the fact that Mollie didn't have a boyfriend for New Year's Eve and under the current situation I was in, we gladly kept the bottle near us. Two bottles of champagne and a mountain of wrapping paper later we went into the dining room for an early dinner. I had never been at a table with so many people! Okay it wasn't that many people but the fact that I couldn't see everyone to the left to me when I was sitting was a new experience.

After dinner Zak, his girlfriend, Mollie, Nathan and I took a short drive to his grandparent's house. This house had been deemed "the farmhouse" and that is exactly what it was. It seemed to look more like a farmhouse than the one we had been at earlier but this was partly due to the surroundings. There were a few sparse old pine trees near the house but past the driveway was a field covered in matted dry grasses that tumbled down into a valley just out of sight. Nathan and Zak gave the city girl a tour of the rustic house while Mollie and I lay down on an old, soft, wooden bed in a room that smelled of antiques.

The ride back into town was quite shorter than I remembered on the way out to the farmhouse. We got back just in time for dessert, but I chose sitting outside on the porch. The mist had been replaced by a cool wind that blew through my fleece every now and again. Considering how overcast it was it seemed unusually warm for the end of December . . . or maybe it was the champagne. I sat in an old wicker loveseat while Zak and Nathan played Frisbee golf, the rules of which I still don't understand, but it looked like something they started a long time ago. Zak's girlfriend came outside and sat down near me still as quiet as before. I tried in vain to start a conversation, but gave up quickly. Instead I choose to quiet my own racing mind. The world I saw out in front of me seemed to be in slow motion. It looked plain and common—another rainy New England Christmas in a small town. I could see the property borders marked by an old log fence and across the yard another weathered house loomed out of the fog. It had huge bare lilac bushes, almost like trees, that created a latticed wall between us. Sporadically a car or truck would slowly drive down the wet street lined with old maple trees, but other than that there was no one around. I felt that if I tried hard enough I could stay in this moment with the wind, the dampness, the grey skies, and the smell of woodstove . . . forever.

We said our goodbyes after the boys finished their game. Everyone got back into their cars and headed home. That Christmas was just another Christmas in Keene, similar to the one before and most likely similar to the ones to follow.

5

Sundays

Carl Printzlau

I toss and turn. Half of my covers are on the hardwood floor next to my bed. The clock at the foot of my bed is blank. I haven't plugged it in since I rearranged my bedroom. I reach down to the floor and rummage through my fallen comforter to find my cell phone. I check the time; it's two thirty, Sunday afternoon. I haven't seen a Sunday morning in months; I'm lucky if I can drag my ass out of bed before one o'clock these days. I slowly swing my tired legs over my bedside. Before I do anything I need a drink. I have a miniature fridge at the end of my bed. I do my best to keep it stocked with Dr. Pepper, but I've been somewhat slacking since I started school. Accordingly, there nothing there. I have to go downstairs.

Downstairs my dog is lying in her Harley Davidson bed. She looks up at me. Her face shows she's been up a while. Her name is Gidget and I only see her on occasion now that I'm off at school. I find myself a cold Dr. Pepper and head back upstairs to my room. She follows me. She loves to follow people. She has a short attention span so usually she will just follow you and then do everything in her power to find something or someone else to follow. She jumps up on my couch and makes herself comfortable; I must be the only one in the house. I ask her how her day has been but she doesn't reply.

It's Sunday, so that means I have school tomorrow, but I don't usually go on Mondays so I'm not too worried about it. I pull up the shades of my oversized windows. The sun is bright but I can tell that it's cold outside. I absolutely hate the winter; it has completely swallowed up my comfort, and has stolen my Sundays. The winter is lonely and cold.

I remember Sundays. They used to be golden and warm and I'd spend them outside on my roof, smoking in the sun. Sundays were our day. I would roll over in the early morning and my half closed eyes would meet hers. Her eyes were always gray blue and always open. My bed was next to my oversized windows then. The sun would pour through these windows and drape blanket upon blanket of warmth, until it was almost too unbearable to sleep. It was my natural alarm clock. Now the shades stay closed for most of the day. When I'm home I usually stick to more artificial forms of light—they tend to stay more consistent.

My Dr. Pepper is half gone, and I start for the bathroom. I turn on the shower so the water can start warming up. I look at myself in the medicine cabinet mirror. My eyes are still half squinting and tiny wrinkles burst from their sides. My hair has gotten long and is knotted from the previous night and my attempts to find the perfect position to sleep. I haven't cut it for months; I used to sit on the roof with my lady and talk about how once it got long she would help me dread it. It's long right now but remains to be dreaded. I suppose the shower is warm enough now so I step in, bringing the rest of my can of Dr. Pepper with me.

I step out of the shower and check my cell phone to see if anyone has called. No one has. It's about three now, early Sunday afternoon. It still doesn't feel like Sunday. I feel too alone for it to be Sunday. I should be sitting at a picnic table, fingers playing with strands of smoke before it leaves with the summer wind. The leaves should be bright with reds and oranges, but they aren't. In fact, there aren't any leaves on the trees at all. There isn't any warm breeze, and there's no her. She was my Sunday excuse. Now there's no need to wake up before the afternoon. I wouldn't know what to do with my time.

I look out my window, clouds cover the sky. My room isn't sheltered anymore. The branches are bare and provide no cover. When the trees are in full foliage they form a twisted wall of lush green and the roof provides a perfect perch for two small tired bodies. I used to spend hours sitting there, smoking and talking. We'd talk about her problems, and how she was handling them. She would talk about how she was different, and that she loved it like that. I would laugh because I liked how different she thought she was, and how very much the same I thought she was. We would talk about movies, my dog, her nephew, and candy. It was a simple relationship, a Sunday relationship.

I cherished my Sundays then as I cherish their memories now, though I suppose at the time the emotion was far more vivid. She was helping me through a hard time, Sunday by Sunday. I was helping keep her grounded; her mind had a habit of finding itself floating off. I needed those moments. We made good companions.

My Dr. Pepper is gone and I'm fully dressed. My dog has left her spot on my couch, most likely looking for something to follow. She's a great dog and I love her. Whenever I really need someone to spend some time with she's more than often there by my side, ready to chill. But after a while, just like my Sunday's she's off, gone, gone to follow something, not for any reason in particular, just for the sake of following it. Maybe she's got some idea where my Sundays up and left to, but probably not, she's just a dog.

I wonder where she went. It was Sunday and I tried calling. She didn't answer; I didn't even get her voicemail. I brushed it off, her phone hardly worked. I tried again a few times. It was Sunday again before I knew it and still nothing. Each Sunday came and passed just as quickly, soon enough I stopped calling. I stopped keeping track of what day it was. Now they come and go, each the same. Different classes, different activities, different people, but each day is the same. I don't much mind.

I take a seat on my couch. This place didn't used to be here, it still feels new. My room was sliding off the rest of the house, so we rebuilt the entire thing. In the process we added a new dormer, and now there is a couch there. Everything seems different now. The trees outside are swaying. I can hear the cold wind nip at the windows and the corners of my bedroom. The clouds are moving fast across the sky. Their shapes are familiar but don't stay the same for more than a moment. I reach down and begin to tie my sneakers.

"Gidget." I hear tiny footsteps heading my way. I throw my feet up to rest on the coffee table I built. My dog jumps up next to me. "You find what you were looking for?" I ask. She doesn't answer. I wonder how much she actually understands. She probably doesn't even know what day it is. "D'you want a treat before I go?" Her tail starts to wag. She understands that; I figured she would.

We both head downstairs. I get her a treat and she carries it in her tiny mouth to her bed. I lock up and head out to my car. It's just as cold as I expected outside; the wind is strong and bites my skin. Short sleeves were a bad call. I start looking at the clouds again, they haven't stopped moving. I can hear geese. They're coming back.

• • •

Writer's Reflection

Of the papers we did, my favorite was my personal essay. It helped that it was about something that meant so much to me, but I think that even if it hadn't, the lessons we learned in class would have helped.

I did what I could to provide imagery that was strong, nothing surreal or mesmerizing; I just tried to be real. For example, the clouds in my essay were very important to me. I mentioned them a few times and I wanted to convey exactly what I remember about watching them in the sky. As they move they form too many shapes to count, and if you look hard enough you can see a picture of them, but then a moment later it's gone, and you have to search for a picture again. The clouds weren't the only imagery I spent some time with, but clouds came up more than once in the final piece.

We also talked about time and its use in writing. With *Sundays* I tried to keep the pace slow but not necessarily dragging. I wanted it to read naturally, and have the story move at the same pace as whoever was reading it. One of the things I did to show the passage of time was my Dr. Pepper. I don't really know if it actually affected how time seemed to pass but it's what I was trying. In the story I change back and forth from action and thought process, so I wanted some fixed object that could act as an hourglass of sorts.

I wanted to end my essay on a light note, because I really hate sad endings. I played around with truth and added the last line about the geese. I don't actually remember if I heard geese, or saw geese, but there were geese in the sky around the time I wrote the paper so I figure it wouldn't be too much of a lie. I used them to pull the story full circle and leave the reader on a more uplifted note. After talking about loneliness and winter, I figured the lines, "I start looking at the clouds again, they haven't stopped moving. I can hear geese. They're coming back" would do the trick.

In this essay I tried hard to find a flow that was my own. I wanted my piece to have a voice that was memorable. I wanted it to stay simple, so that the actual reading of the piece would compliment and let the feelings and emotion behind it come through clearly.

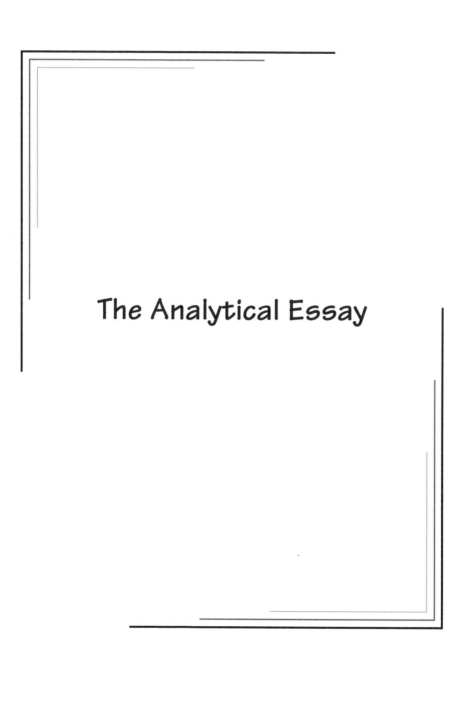

The Analytical Essay

6

Control and Conquest Won't Goewey

Erin Harrison

In his essay "'Careful, You May Run out of Planet': SUVs and the Exploitation of the American Myth," David Goewey argues that "the sport utility vehicle is a full-fledged myth machine, symbolically incorporating many of America's ideological values and contradictions within its several tons of heavy metal" (112). The American obsession with exploration and conquest is latent in our history and a large part of our present. In some cases, wars have been started over the United States' efforts to expand. Goewey's thesis is that the Ford Explorer and the Jeep Cherokee symbolize the American obsession of conquering the frontier while other sport utility names follow in their footsteps of symbolizing the historical American obsession with control, conquest, and essentially expansion. However, Goewey's contention does not account for the fact that the American obsession with conquest will continue into the future. Although our past and present are already plagued with the American ideology of conquest and control, the future is undoubtedly doomed to share the same fate.

This American infatuation with conquest and control is evident in our past. As stated by Goewey, sport utility vehicle names such as the Jeep Wrangler and Cherokee reflect the conquest motif saturating our past. The Wrangler refers to the glorified role of the Wild West cowboys that serve as the basis of hundreds of 19th-century dime novels. In actuality, "long hours, low pay, and hazardous work discouraged many older ranch hands from applying [to be a cowboy]. At odds with the lonely, dirty, and often boring cowboy life were the exploits of the mythic frontier cowboy, glamorized by the eastern press" (Boyer 377). The life of an authentic cowboy usually consisted of grueling, dangerous work, which explains why this way of life slowly died out as farming and industrialization expanded into the western United States. Similarly, the Jeep Cherokee glorifies an aspect of history Americans have chosen to cover up. This durable vehicle that can supposedly take on any terrain is a reflection of our horrible treatment of the Cherokee tribe in the 1820s and 1830s when the U.S. government forced these innocent people to leave their homes. When President Andrew Jackson discussed the removal of the Cherokee people with Congress, he said, "Our conduct towards these people" would reflect "on our national character" (Cave 1332). Consistent throughout history, our national character has been to expand and take control of land at any expense. However, Americans tend to ignore the truth and covered up details of the past while focusing on the victory of conquest they associate with names like Wrangler and Cherokee.

Presently, cars that promise exploration and the conquest of nature reflect the focus of American ideology. The Ford Motor Company alone has the Explorer, Expedition, Excursion, and Escape to symbolize America's fascination with conquest and expansion. There are also the Honda Odyssey and Chevy Trailblazer to further prove the American obsession. Again Goewey suggests that "capable of handling the roughest terrain . . . much of the appeal of SUVs is their promise of providing access to the farthest reaches of the globe" (119). Each car advertisement displays the car in an exotic landscape obviously of another country or on the top of a U.S. mountain we stole from a people conquered two centuries ago. The suggestion of these ads is that there is no mountain, jungle, rapid flow of water, environmental challenge, or culture that one cannot conquer when in the vehicle. Such limitlessness gives the car owner a feeling of power and control, which again is a reflection of the American ideology of conquest and control.

Coincidental to the attitude of control and conquest is our present involvement in the War on Terror. Originating as a war to defend our role as a world leader, invulnerable to any foreign influence or terrorist persuasion, the War on Terror proves the American ideology of control and conquest. Other countries reacted to the attack on United States soil as an "attack on the world's most powerful country or, as many have argued, an attack on civilization itself" ("Seeing the World Anew" 19). Throughout history, several countries have been the target of terrorism. Although tragic, these attacks were viewed as a normal part of a violent world. Some of these attacks were even funded by the United States such as in the case of the CIA-funded assassination of the Dominican ruler El Jefe. Several United States embassies have been bombed on foreign soil, but such attacks have not rendered a reaction as globally strong as the response to September 11, 2001. When terrorists attacked the United States on home soil, the world saw it as implausible. As "America—and indeed the world—stopped still to watch what seemed like a horrific movie that no one ever wanted to see? it became apparent that the United States was not invulnerable" (Tyson et al. 1). The world opinion was that the United

States was almighty, the one who did the conquering and was never attacked. The September 11th attacks threatened the United States image as a world power, and thus when the roles of power reversed, the United States reacted strongly and put themselves back into a position of control. To defend the American reputation, the United States went to war and thus perpetuated the ideology of control and conquest while also fulfilling the expectations of surrounding countries.

As the War on Terror progressed, and the United States attempted to rid the world of terror and re-established itself as a world leader, the American ideology of control and conquest again arose. However noble our intentions were in the beginning of the war, the present focus of the war seems to have changed to the same Cold War agenda of democratization. Yet again, Americans have gone beyond their own realm of power in an effort to force our ideology onto another people. Although Islamic extremists bombed the United States in an effort to end the spread of Western ideals and stop the American culture from destroying their own, the reaction to the Islamic extremists' efforts have thus far been the opposite. The American obsession with control and conquest is obvious with magazines like the *Economist* exclaiming that "one big reason the Americans gave for the war in Iraq was to bring democracy to the Iraqis" ("First Give" 43). Through the conversion of the Iraqi government to democracy, the United States can more easily work with Iraqis in foreign issues such as trade and capitalism. The United States will also acquire access to certain Iraqi natural resources. One of which is oil, a very ironic resource to gain access to since the names of our inefficient fuel-consuming SUVs symbolize the control obsessed ideology. The American ideology of conquest and control may be symbolized in our car names, but it is proven in our actions of conquest-motivated war.

Elaborating upon the global expectations of the United States as protector of the world, the United States was also expected to intervene and aid Indonesia after the tsunami. Other countries automatically expected the United States to be the first to give aid and also to be the largest donator of monetary aid. However, the United States appeared to hesitate in sending aid, and many countries were shocked to see this known control-crazy country show reluctance in being present in the affairs of another country. When Australian volunteers arrived in Indonesia two days after the tsunami, the world wondered what the United States was waiting for. On January 2, "the carrier group the USS Abraham Lincoln arrived; it was made up of 1,500 personnel, 23 ships and about 100 aircraft—helicopters and fixed-wing aircraft. A fully equipped hospital ship, the USNS Mercy, arrived on February 2" (Yew 39). The United States was one of the last countries to bring support, and the world saw this as not only out of character but greedy as well. Because Americans have a history of inviting themselves to help other countries, the world expects them to live up to their reputation and thus the American ideology is perpetuated through these worldwide expectations. The fact that the United States had to travel the farthest distance to give aid did not occur to other countries. The world only saw a power-hungry country delay in giving aid. Therefore, the American ideology of control and conquest is so embedded in the American past that it is expected in its present and probably in its future as well.

Our past and present actions confirm the American preoccupation with control and conquest. In fact, our aggressive influence in other countries has ensured that the American ideology will live on. Our future is doomed to be abundant with events that have conquest motives, and thus will probably be latent with the same symbolic consumer products. Soon there will be a day when the car companies simply avoid symbolism and just name their cars the Jeep Islamic Conqueror or the Ford Jungle Destroyer. Americans have no intention of giving up their ideology of exploration, control, and conquest.

The American ideology of control and conquest will prevail through time for it is in our nature. Not only do Americans strive to survive but we also have the unquenchable thirst to expand. Our history has proven these desires, and instead of learning from the destruction we have caused in our greediness, Americans ignore their blunders and glorify their actions by naming vehicles after their mistakes. This belief of infallibility allows the American ideology to continue and thus it will inevitably exist through future generations. Plus, with other countries expecting the United States to involve themselves in foreign affairs, any inactivity or hesitation by the United States is questioned and criticized. The vicious cycle of explore and destroy will continue until the day Americans finally decide to accept their mistakes and rebuild from them while simultaneously shocking the world with a new image.

Works Cited

Boyer, Paul. *The Enduring Vision: A History of the American People*. 2nd ed. Lexington, MA: D.C. Heath and Company, 1995.

Cave, Alfred A. "Abuse of Power: Andrew Jackson and the Indian Removal Act of 1830." *The Historian* 65 (2003): 1330-1355.

"First Give Them Power of a Kind, Then Let's Discuss Democracy." *Economist* 22 (November 2003): 43.

Goewey, David. "'Careful. You May Run out of Planet': SUVs and the Exploitation of the American Myth." *Signs of Life in the USA: Readings on Popular Culture for Writers*. 4th ed. Sonia Maasik and Jack Solomon. Boston: Bedford/St. Martin's, 2003. 112-121.

"Seeing the World Anew." *Economist* 27 (October 2001): 19.

Tyson, Ann Scott, et al. "From London to Los Angeles, the World Stood Still." *Christian Science Monitor* 93.202 (2001):1.

Yew, Lee Kuan. "Competition in Compassion." *Forbes* 175.8 (2005): 39.

7

Deceitful Advertising

Matthew J. Connors

In the 1950s, 60s, and 70s advertisements were easy identifiable. But classical advertising of the mid-twentieth century is dead. Classical advertisement like those containing catchy jingles and celebrity endorsements are long gone. In modern society advertisements that are easily recognizable to the general public are not effective and classical advertising are mainstream, too easily spotted, and therefore too easily dismissed. Advertisements are no longer the sole medium of introducing and distributing consumer goods. Advertisers have turned the once neutral agents of the media into necessary unsuspecting actors of their selling machine. Advertising in modern society has become more deceitful than ever before, being integrated to the detriment of news, television, entertainment, and politics.

The media world is comprised of the largest corporations in the world such as Disney, AOL Time-Warner, and Viacom International. Each of these corporations own a broadcasting company, a movie production studio, and at least one company that produces consumer goods. Due to widespread ownership, a news company will advertise another program belonging to their parent network by highlighting it as a news story. David Colander, advertising and economics professor at Middlebury College, identifies this form of advertising as a combination of an advertisement and news editorial, thus the name as advertorials (315). An example of an advertorial was the amount of coverage of the anniversary of Pearl Harbor on ABC's World News Tonight; the coverage often mentioned the upcoming release of Disney's new movie *Pearl Harbor*. It comes as no surprise that Disney owns ABC. This practice of advertorials is deceitful to the viewing public because the news no longer reports news but rather a related synopsis of their parent companies latest venture. It is detrimental to the news industry because it detracts from the credibility of the news organization.

Television since its inception has been littered with advertisements during commercial breaks. But today the commercial advertisement isn't just for the commercial break. The MTV network is actually one long continuous advertisement. For example, the MTV program TRL plays a select number of music videos with some commentary in between from a stylish host and the occasional musical guest. Everything on this program is an advertisement. The music videos are advertisements for the musicians; the clothing worn by the host is nothing but the newest fashions and is clearly shown on camera; the musical guests who visit the show plug their upcoming releases and that is all without considering the plethora of ads that can be seen in the backdrop of their Time Square studio. The entire network is a misleading advertisement because no matter what their viewers watch they are exposed to some kind of advertisement, and that is excluding actual commercial breaks.

Corporations are not only controlling advertorials on television but in newspapers as well. All of the major corporations command massive public relations departments whose efforts are on behalf of their employer's agendas. In the United States, the 170,000 public relations employees whose job it is to manipulate news, public opinion, and public policy in the interests of their employers outnumber news reporters by 40,000 (Robbins 138). Richard Robbins in his study, *Global Problems and the Culture of Capitalism,* discovers that almost 40 percent of the news content of a typical U.S. newspaper originates as public relations press releases (138). Robbins expands with the example that "more than half the news stories in the *New York Times* are based solely on corporate press releases, which are often related to some form a profit venture" (138). So not only do corporations pedal advertisements via their own news outlets, but also make their press releases, which are a type of advertisement, so newsworthy that newspapers feel the need to print stories about them. This method of advertising is deceitful to newspaper readers and the newspapers themselves. Readers are not conscious to the fact that they are reading a glorified advertisement, and newspapers are not aware that they are even printing free advertising. But the news industry is not the only victim of such inconspicuous advertisements.

Short films are viewed for entertainment by thousands of people everyday on the Internet or as "shorts" before a feature film. Advertisers have taken these short films and created Advertainment (Jhally). These mini films are very entertaining and exciting, seeming similar to any short film but at that same time convey an underlining promotion a product that is often related to the main theme of the film. For example, Mitsubishi motors recently spent $25 million dollars on a 15-minute short film showcasing a car chase between a Mitsubishi Eclipse and Toyota Camry. The short film does not have many similarities with a television commercial; it has no voiceover, no information about financing the car, or anything of that nature. The film instead cuts between the two cars, quickly showing the Mitsubishi logo any time the car is shown, where as the Toyota logo is painted over to make the car generic. The film is found on Atom Films web site, a web site that showcases short independent films. The deception in this advertisement is two-fold. First the advertisement is found on a web site that viewers are not expecting to see advertisements, thus they are totally oblivious to the fact that what they are watching is an advertisement. The second deception is borderline illegal because the advertisement can be construed as subliminal messaging. Subliminal messaging is an illegal practice in which someone is exposed to a motion picture or TV show that contains single slides of a message, such as an advertisement, and has proven to be highly effective in getting the viewer to comply with whatever the message may be. Advertising has not only saturated viewable entertainment with advertainments, but also entertainment events.

Consumers across America go out every Friday and Saturday night to music concerts. Advertisers having noticed this trend began implementing the advertainment strategy into the concert scene. In the PBS documentary, *Merchants of Cool*, thousands of young adults are invited to what they think is just a hip-hop. However, the Coca-Cola company product, Sprite, is putting on the concert. The concert is decorated with Sprite logos and flashy green lighting; the entire event looks like it could be taking place inside a 20 oz. bottle of Sprite. While these young people are under the impression that they are merely getting a free night out at a hip-hop concert, they are actually being inundated with advertisements for Sprite. Advertisement is not the only means for advertisers to reach consumers.

Cinema-goers have been keen to product placement in films for years because of countless examples where the camera lingers for too long over a logo before shifting back to the main action. But product placement has gone attained a whole new way according to *BBC Magazine*'s Jonathan Duffy, author of *Well Placed*, "now, more than 50 years after Hollywood wised up to the fact that companies will pay to have their brands featured within the narrative of a movie, but advertisers have begun to extend the principle to formats such as books, pop songs, videos and computer games." These new generation product placements not only catch the consumers completely off-guard, but also can be very effective. Most consumers are not anticipating an advertisement to be presented to them when they read a book and if the consumer is enjoying the book then they will associate the advertisement with the enjoyed book.

Politics was an area that was widely untouched by advertisers until the last twenty years. In recent years however advertisers have found their way into politics to ensure not only that they have the ear of political powers but also that their product or name is associated with the political powers. Alexander Cohen in "Bush Lobbyist" reports this about President George W. Bush:

> Lobbyists for Ferris & Glovsky, People PC, Sony, AT&T, and Clear Channel fell under the senator's purview. Each lobbyist became a contributor making donations ranging from more than a $100,000 to $10 million to Bush's campaign over the years.

Big corporations would shell out huge sums of money for nothing. Each company in return received hours of free television advertising in the form of campaign coverage. This advertising, which aired on national television, came when President Bush used an AT&T cell-phone or Sony television, or when he stood in front of the Clear Channel banner at political rallies. So when Joe Average American turns on the television to see the president's speech he is not only listening to the speech but is also looking at advertisements for President Bush's sponsors.

While advertisers could argue that there is nothing wrong with their new tactics of deceitful advertising, saying it is just a more sophisticated way to sell products, that may be less forthcoming because people are smart enough that they don't need to explicitly mention that "this is a commercial." But in fact it would be good for people to be aware of what they are watching because with the deceitful policy of advertising today people can't tell if they are watching, reading, attending, or voting for something totally unrelated instead of absorbing an advertisement.

Works Cited

Cohen, Alexander. "Bush Lobbyist." *The Center for Public Integrity.* 15 Apr. 2005. <http://www.publicintegrity.org/bop2004/report.aspx?aid=273&sid=200>.

Colander, David. *Macro Economics & Advertising.* 5th ed. New York: McGraw Hill & Irwin, 2004.

Duffy, Jonathan. "Well Placed." *BBC News Magazine* 30 Mar. 2005.

"Merchants of Cool." *Frontline.* PBS, WGBH, Boston, 2004.

Jhally, Sut. "How TV Works." *CML: Center for Media Literacy.* 9 Feb. 2005. http://www.medialit.org/reading_room/article83.html>.

Robbins, Richard. *Global Problems and the Culture of Capitalism.* New York: McGraw Hill & Irwin, 1999.

8

MTV Food

Lindsey Fitzpatrick

Celebrities in America are so famous that we couldn't make them more famous if we wanted to. They are constantly integrating themselves in so many aspects of our lives. Americans are extremely influenced by celebrities and in many cases they even take on the role as decision makers for our actions and our lifestyle choices. When deciding on whether or not to change our hair color we will consult the latest gossip magazine and see what hair color Brittany Spears is sporting these days. When Professor Susan Boon of the University of Calgary conducted a survey consisting of 200 undergraduate college students it was shocking that "a whopping 60 percent admitted that an idol had influenced their attitudes and personal values, including their work ethic and views on morality" (Bennett). Celebrities are slowly destroying the word unique because we are emulating them at a rapid pace, giving up the qualities that make each one of us an individual. It seems that this ridiculous behavior would be obvious and shunned, but it is a perpetual problem that we do not desire to put an end to. On the contrary, the entertainment industry is feeding our desires to further duplicate celebrity lifestyles. Specifically, Music Television is creating shows that devote time to giving fans a taste of what it is to be a celebrity. With shows such as *Make My Video*, *I Want a Famous Face*, and *Real World* who knows when a fan can stay a fan without losing their individualistic features. MTV is a television station that feeds a fan's desire to emulate their favorite celebrity and ultimately robs them of their individuality.

Viewers of the MTV channel are fans desiring to look just like their favorite celebrity. Even in Music Television's early years, producers of this station were dedicated to satisfying a fan's desire to perfectly match a star's style. In one case, when Madonna released her third album in the fall of 1986, her record company along with MTV promoted a fan look-a-like contest. The contest asked for fans to submit their take on Madonna's newest video, "True Blue." The winner of this *Make My Video* contest would receive a $25,000 check that would be presented live on MTV (Lewis 173). The producers of MTV realized that Madonna had a large fan base and that her fans would respond to the challenge. According to Lisa Lewis, author of *Gender Politics and MTV*, "thousands of viewers submitted tapes" (206). Because of the many fans who desired to look like their favorite celebrity, Madonna's *Make My Video* contest was a success.

As innocent and simple as a look-a-like contest seems, MTV had a strategy in airing this show. Lewis states that, MTV was "using style imitation as their preferred mode of response, the girl fans became highly visible at concerts and shopping malls, on movie and television screens, so much so that they became news on national television" (174). With all of their publicity, Madonna fans were just that, a Madonna fan. That title meant the loss of their own unique sense of style and a complete acquirement of their idol, Madonna's fashion. Instead of fans being individualists who just happen to like the same music, they were a cult-like fan base that dressed in exactly the same manner. MTV created a show exhibiting their power to satisfy a fan's want to look like a celebrity that they idolize and at the same time rob this viewer of his or her uniqueness. With the realization of how fan's desire to look like their favorite celebrities, MTV created a program that was devoted to a fan forgetting about his or her individuality and acquiring a celebrity's qualities, in this case Madonna's features.

From seemingly innocent fashion duplications to the more drastic measures that fans have gone to recently, MTV is creating shows that exploit a fan's desire to emulate a celebrity. Last year, MTV created a show called *I Want a Famous Face*. The title is pretty self-explanatory, but the show takes a person who wants to completely resemble their favorite celebrity to a plastic surgeon that will perform the necessary procedures to give the fan the famous face they so desperately desire. MTV gives a description of the show saying, "Whether it's a Pamela Anderson wanna be or a Janet Jackson hopeful, their goals are not just to look differently, but to look exactly like their favorite stars" (*I Want*). Fans want to completely resemble a celebrity, not just partially. The fact that people will go to the extent to change their physical appearance in a drastic way to physically duplicate their favorite celebrities is frightening, and almost more frightening is that there is a show starring this type of procedure. Elizabeth, a viewer of the show, comments on a specific episode featuring a young woman desiring to look like Kate Winslet, "I really felt MTV was irresponsible in supporting her in that. But to do otherwise would be to undermine their reason for existing—to glorify the lives of the beautiful people and suck us in with our own desires to be like them" ("I Want"). Here, Elizabeth emphasizes how awful it is that a show like this is in existence and how MTV truly does create this show to feed a fan's desire to emulate the famous.

As more fans have these procedures done, the farther from individuals they become. Because MTV is giving fans the opportunity to alter their physique to represent that of the desired celebrity, the fan is ultimately being robbed of their unique characteristics. This idea is explained in the article "In the Cut" by Dennis Cass who states that, "conventional wisdom says that popular culture corrupts one's idea of the self." Cass believes shows such as *I Want a Famous Face* take away who you once were. MTV is feeding a fan's desire to emulate their favorite celebrity by broadcasting this type of show. As a result, a fan's previous identity is taken away and replaced with the physical features of the celebrity they wished to be. MTV, a television station, has created yet another show that feeds a fan's craving to look just like their favorite celebrity which has robbed them of their individuality.

MTV will also fill a fan's desire for, what I like to call, bottled fame that only lasts for ten minutes to achieve the level of fame that their favorite celebrities experience. With a show such as *Real World*, participants will be viewed on TV for a few months at a time and will actually be "famous" for about, realistically, a month after the show has aired. Viewers of these shows are drawn in because they feel as if they are watching real people that they could possibly be friends with. The author of *Media & Culture* describes how a viewer of a reality show like *Real World* is refreshed to see an average person on TV with his statement:

> . . . in a high-tech age where people feel increasingly cut off from the powerful and excluded from big-money, two-party politics, it's a novelty to see ordinary people take the stage for a little fame and a little power. We identify. (Campbell, Fabos, and Martin 150)

The realistic nature of *Real World* helps viewers feel connected to each "character" and they become attached. When the show airs its final episode, it is upsetting to let these people that you feel you have come to know, leave. MTV won't let you be sad for long though, after a week a new *Real World* will premier and you will fall in love with new characters. What happens to participants of previous seasons? They go from instant fame to performing an all too common disappearance act. Fans of celebrities see this as their chance to achieve some level of fame. The article entitled "So You Wanna Get on The Real World?" describes the desire for instant fame and how MTV satisfies this craving:

Most of us have it in us somewhere—that voyeuristic, self-proclaimed movie star just waiting for the right time to jump out into the limelight. And *The Real World* is just the place to do it. After all, with no acting experience to speak of, you can parlay your 15 minutes of fame into a full-fledged third-rate career.

Although coated with sarcasm, the article proves that MTV has created this show because they realize a fan's desire to reach the level of fame that their favorite celebrity encompasses.

But how does the desire for fame take away our individuality? If you have watched even just a few of the seasons of *Real World* you have noticed that there are certain characters that continuously pop up. There always seems to be a gay guy, the macho man, a beautiful girl, etc. I even found a quiz titled, "Which Real World Character Are You?" I already know that if I were to take this quiz or apply to be on the show I would be shown as the innocent girl next door because I haven't had to overcome any serious issues in my life. Instead of being viewed as the Lindsey that I am I would be displayed as someone I'm not. The article, "So You Wanna Get on *The Real World?*" reinforces the fact that there are molds people are squeezed into for the show with the statement, "MTV casting agents seem to have developed a tried-and-true formula for creating chemistry (good and bad). You'll notice that many of the selected cast have such strong personality types, that they seem to be living cartoon characters." When you go into the casting interviews with MTV agents you must conform to a certain mold, even if this is not really who you are, to be on the cast of this show. *The Real World* is squeezing each person desiring to have instant fame into character molds, completely shedding participants of their individuality that they previously owned. The result is a cast of a show that is molded into characters and robbed of individuality. MTV realizes the fact that fans want to acquire the fame that their favorite celebrities have and they will create a show that feeds this hunger.

Being an average and avid viewer of MTV I realize that you must take all shows with a grain of salt and enjoy its entertainment value. These shows are sheer entertainment, but what seems obvious to me now is that the shows discussed are targeted to celebrity fanatics because of the desire to be just like the celebrities that consume our lives. We want to dress like them, look like them, and be admired just like they are and MTV has capitalized upon this exact idea. The producers realize that fans want to be like their favorite celebrities so they have created shows that feed this addiction. MTV has become a fan's food when he or she is hungry for celebrity fashion, beauty, and fame. This seems like MTV is just giving a fan what they are asking for, but is it right that with these shows they are slowly taking away a fan's individuality? Whether it is morally right or not, MTV is a television station devoted to feeding a fan's desire for the celebrity lifestyle and in a gradual process they are taking with them unique qualities that the fan once had.

Works Cited

Bennett, Courtney. "Fan Club Confessions: Teens Underestimate Influence of Celebrity Idols." Starstruck. 2 May 2005 <http://www.psychologytoday.com>.

Cass, Dennis. "In the Cut." 14 April 2004. 3 May 2005 http://slate.msn.com>.

Fabos, Bettina and Christopher R. Martin. Boston: Bedford/St. Martin's, 2002. 150-189.

I Want a Famous Face. 10 April 2005 http://www.mtv.com.

"I Want a Famous Face." Online posting. 8 Apr. 2004. <hugoboy.typepad.com>.

Lewis, Lisa A. Gender Politics and MTV. Philadelphia: Temple UP, 1990. 173-213.

·So You Wanna Get on the Real World? 2 May 2005 <http://www.soyouwanna.com>.

"Television and the Power of Visual Culture." Media & Culture. Comp. Richard Campbell,

Which Real World Character Are You? 1 May 2005 <http://www.java.alloy.com>.

9

Birkenstock Shoes

Amanda Diegel

Throughout the history of marketing in the United States, certain products have become the representation of specific ideals and lifestyles. At the same time, many of these particular bonds between product and ideals have become exploited and disintegrated by the transition of the product from underground acceptance to mass appeal. Birkenstock shoes have been subject to both of these phenomenon since its first inception in the United States, where they have come to represent specific ideals about the emerging hippie subculture in the late 1960s and recently have become desired by the general public. Through understanding how Birkenstock has been adapted by this hippie subculture, the relationship the company established in sharing its mutual beliefs, and how it therefore came to represent this particular lifestyle, one can see why the growing popularity of the shoe over time and the recent burst in Birkenstock knockoffs have begun to change the nature of the company, diminish the authenticity of the original shoe, and ultimately sever its semiotic ties.

The series of events involving the targeted market and response to the shoe following Birkenstock's introduction to the United States in 1966 has come to etch the strong association of the shoe with the environmentally concerned, hippie subculture that many Americans continue to make today. Responsible for first exposing the 200-year-old shoe company to the American people was Margaret Fraser, who stumbled upon the company while traveling through her native country. Fraser purchased a pair of Birkenstocks in Germany in hopes of alleviating the chronic foot problems she assumed were from the poor form of generic footwear. She became so impressed with the shoes' comfort, as Birkenstock originated the radical concept of using cork soles to mold to the owners foot, that she eventually began importing small orders of the shoe to the United States and selling them near her home in the San Francisco area. Birkenstocks were originally sold discretely in health food stores, and the positive response from that particular crowd consequently created a stereotype of the shoe belonging to an "earthy-crunchy" environment. As Corporate Design Foundation asserts, "back in the San Francisco Bay area, however, Fraser found that traditional shoe stores considered the wide curved-sole sandals simply too ugly to carry, so she peddled them to health food stores where the granola-and-sprouts crowd welcomed their orthopedic, eco-friendly design" ("From Hippie to Hip" 1).

What drew this emerging hippie subculture to Birkenstock during the time of its first introduction in the United States was that the shoes were the physical manifestation of their newly forming, radical environmentally friendly and anti-consumerist philosophies. Unlike most plastic and rubber based shoes, the soles are composed of cork, a widely known renewable resource that promoted recycling and sustainable lifestyles this particular group of society identified with. Although the shoe was expensive, it could be repaired easily and repeatedly by cobblers for minimal costs, which unwittingly brought the economy back to skilled craftsmen and away from the newly emerging, large corporate monopolies, even if only on a small scale. Pioneers in this hippie subculture celebrated the shoe for these factors in that it appropriately conformed to their lifestyle by leaving less to want, less to accumulate, and less to waste as a shoe. Likewise, Leslie Brokaw alludes in her article "Feet Don't Fail Me Now" that the shoe was adapted by these hippies because to the "practical minded folk hopelessly untuned to the fashion world, the leather strapped, molded cork based concoctions looked fine, felt fine, and were the casual shoe of impassioned choice" (1).

In response to this seemingly universal acceptance of such a minority of American culture to its shoe, Birkenstock incorporated the beliefs of their zealous buyers in their company policy, thereby creating a powerful bond between maker and buyer that further tied the shoe to this rising subculture. Sharing the same environmental beliefs, Birkenstock went on to initiate the Birkenstock Green Team during the late 1960s, whose mission statement still appropriately states that "as a company we strive to: educate ourselves and associates about environmental issues, minimize consumption and re-use when possible, and purchase recycled products from environmentally responsible companies" ("Birkenstock Green Team" 1). The company continued to advertise solely on word of mouth, which greatly pleased its customers in their adamant rejection of the consumerist, advertisement driven world around them. This created an image of the company that set it apart from traditional shoe stores, which many belonging to this subculture identified with as they were similarly set apart from conforming ideas of society. In a win-win situation, the owners of the sandals rejoiced the tip off between economy and environment and the company prided itself on what many would consider a drawback of less shipping, packaging, and inventory. Birkenstock became in the realm of consumerism what hippies were as a subculture of society.

As this hippie subculture began fading out in the middle to later seventies, Birkenstock shoes held strong to its once flourishing ideals in the United States and continued selling its shoes in a competitively void market; its semiotic ties to the hippie philosophies helped continue the company's meager, yet self-satisfying growth. The purchasers of Birkenstock shoes were still often those riding on the nostalgia of such a radical era, one which psychologist William Partridge defined, among many other factors, the era's prominent values of "isolation and independence from a larger society, experimentation, and dependency upon esoteric information" (67). Birkenstock shoes were still in many ways the symbol of these values. Much like the people of this timeframe, the shoe remained for quite some time isolated and independent from the realm of consumerism and the sea of brand name, generic, and discount shoe companies. In terms of experimentation, Birkenstock was the living proof of successful alternatives to mass production and flimsily made products. Most defining to the company, Birkenstock relentlessly pushed the esoteric view of environmental conservation through propaganda via footwear. These three factors insinuating the nature of the company, coupled with the basic efficiency of the shoe, caused it to ultimately represent a simple, consumerism free lifestyle that became destroyed later by society's gradual acceptance and sudden burst of popularity in recent years. The first step in the progression of popularity in Birkenstock shoes occurred when future subcultures of society, identifying with similar ideals to the hippie subculture, continued to wear these shoes. Ultimately, this fed to the masses as an advertisement and created a sudden shift in popularity when the general society began accepting and emulating these future subcultures. *The Saint James Encyclopedia of Popular Cultures* accurately depicts this transition of the shoe from one subculture to the next in claming, "countering an association with Deadheads, the hippies, and then grunge rockers, who favored the shoes, and their links to elicit drugs, as well as women who don't shave their legs, Birkenstock featured hip young urbans" (Pendergast 152). The grunge era reinforced some of the associations Birkenstock had made with counter cultures of society, yet when grunge became popular so did many of its fashions. Birkenstocks were no exception. According to *The New York Times*, the company sold more shoes in this era between 1992 and 1994 than it did in the last twenty years before it (Pendergast 153). Around this exact time appeared the birth of Birkenstock knockoffs, which, coupled with this sudden explosion of popularity in the shoe, have come to alter the company approaches to marketing, strip the shoe of its authenticity, and weaken its semiotic ties.

The first thing knockoff Birkenstock shoes accomplished was forcing the company to change from a laid-back, detached company to a capitalist company, which broke the established association between this company and anti-consumerism. Pitted against the competing version of itself that was offered at much cheaper prices in knockoff shoes, Birkenstock had no choice but to become an active capitalist company and vie for its products amongst other shoe companies. By 1990, knockoff shoes were already sold in Kmart, and Birkenstock responded by launching national advertisements, creating relationships between retail stores, and updating product designs. They now offer "some 500 shoe products, sold through 200 licensed independent retailers, as well as its own brand name stores" (Brokaw 1). Birkenstock completely changed its original, meager profiting company into that of a booming industrialist moneymaker, and the change is sourly ironic. However, this was only the first negative effect of Birkenstock knockoffs.

Along with altering the connotation of the company, Birkenstock knockoffs have also recently threatened the authenticity of the original shoe. Philosopher Walter Benjamin's discerning argument about authenticity holds very real life examples with the crisis of Birkenstock shoes, as he states that:

> The presence of the original is the prerequisite to the concept of authenticity. . . . The technique of reproduction detaches the reproduced object from the domain of tradition . . . By making many reproductions, it substitutes a plurality of copies for a unique existence. And in permitting the reproduction to meet the beholder or listener in his own particular situation, it reactivates the object reproduced. These two processes lead to a tremendous shattering of tradition which is the obverse of the contemporary crisis and renewal of mankind (147).

Birkenstocks shoes, although a vocation and not a work of art, are currently facing this exact process of shattering traditions. Once the original shoe pure in symbolism of hippie ideals, it is now undergoing a detachment from its semiotic ties to independence, experimentation, and esoteric information.

Each of these three aforementioned factors of the hippie subculture are indeed loosing their intimate connections with the shoe as a result of Birkenstock knockoffs. Where Birkenstock once related to this subculture through its independence from consumerism, it is now a prominent and profitable company. The argument of experimentation applying to the Birkenstock Company as an alternative to mass production and poorly made shoes became inapplicable upon its merging into the realm of capitalism and the existence of knockoffs that many people cannot discriminate from the original. Lastly, the esoteric viewpoint of environmental concern is losing its meaning and association with the shoe amidst the abundance of knockoff shoes that do not carry this message. The absence of this belief in the knockoff shoes creates a population of owners that are now unaware or unconcerned with such passionate views.

Decades after its first inception into the United States, Birkenstock shoes are facing an inevitable and helpless battle against the transgression into the consumer market. The shoe that has come to favorably represent a low maintenance, environmentally-friendly hippie discourse that promoted independence, experimentation, and esoteric views, is now being reduced to a trendy fashion statement. What was once raw and ignored in the fashion world has now become sought out by a variety of people, many probably unaware of the deep seeded implications of the shoe, and therefore its strong sense of authenticity is fading. For a shoe that has been shaped to embody assertive ideals to a particular group, the newfound popularity of its rebel insinuation is its worst enemy yet.

Works Cited

Benjamin, Walter. "The Work of Art in the Age of Mechanical Reproduction." *Walter Benjamin: Selected Writings, Vol. 3, 1935-1938.* Belnap Press: New York, 2002.

Brokaw, Leslie. "Feet Don't Fail Me Now." *Inc.* (May 94), 70.

"From Hippie to Hip: Birkenstock Goes Urban." *Journal of Business and Design.* 1995.

Corporate Design Issue, Volume 9 Number 1. 14 April 2004. <http://www.cdf.org/91index.html>.

Partridge, William L. *The Hippie Ghetto: The Natural History of a Subculture.* Holt, Rhinehart, and Winston, Inc: New York, 1973.

Pendergast, Sarah and Pendergast, Tom. Comp. *St. James Encyclopedia of Pop Culture*. Detroit: St. James Press, 1999.

"The Birkenstock Green Team." 1997. *Alta Vista*. 24 November 1997. <http://www.birkenstock.com/greenteam.html>.

10

Livestrong . . . Without the Bracelet

Shaun Moore

As Lance Armstrong pedaled past the finish line, winning his sixth consecutive victory of the Tour De France cycling competition, viewers saw a hero who fought his way through cancer and came out a survivor. Yet their eyes were glued to something else . . . a vibrant and appealing yellow wristband with the slogan "Livestrong" engraved on it. In 1996, Armstrong was ranked the top pro cyclist in the world, but in the height of his career, Lance was diagnosed with cancer and was promised less than a fifty percent chance of survival. He struggled, fought hard, and won his battle with cancer, and as a result, Armstrong became a key figure in supporting a cause for cancer (Capitol Sports).

In 1998, Armstrong teamed up with Nike to produce the Livestrong bracelets. The primary meaning behind these bracelets was to support cancer survivors, those who lost their lives to cancer, but more importantly, to raise money for a possible cure. About a month later, young adults and teenagers everywhere were asking where they could purchase their own, some not even knowing the true meaning behind them. I purchased a Livestrong bracelet for the right reason; to support a cause for cancer because both my mother and her brother once had cancer, but they were lucky, they won their battle. I had a reason to support cancer and to wear this bracelet, but I soon noticed how many were wearing them for appeal, wearing them for the wrong reason. Quickly other celebrities and athletes began to wear them, as well as huge political giants such as John Kerry. These bracelets soon became a status symbol for young adults and celebrities alike.

Other companies, as well as political campaigns, quickly took note of how something this simple and incredibly cheap could go so far in producing a large capital for their business. Many companies came out with bracelets like the Nike Livestrong bracelets, some to raise money for a cause, while others were produced because consumers desired them. Some companies fed off of the emotions of the consumers and used this as a tool to create more business for their company. As a result of this cultural phenomenon, thirty-one other forms of the bracelet are now being sold, pedaling down the same path the Livestrong bracelet has smoothly paved (Collector's Paradise). Yet these bracelets are transforming the inherent meaning the Livestrong bracelet proposed.

The Livestrong bracelet was once a heartfelt reason to support such an important cause, but is now merely a fashion article one wears to increase his or her appeal to society. Cancer is a paramount issue that should not be made into a form of capitalization by greedy advertisers and bandwagon consumers. However, the Nike Livestrong bracelet and others like it, have become a symbol of status for the young and rich alike, offering false dignity, respect, personal financial profit and empowerment to all of those who give into its marketed appeal.

Many individuals who wear the Livestrong bracelet may know the true meaning behind it, but they choose to wear it simply because their friends all have one, their favorite athletes wear them, and politicians endorse them. Chris McCoy, journalist for the North Carolina State University's newspaper entitled *Technician*, offers his input as to why people everywhere are now wearing these bracelets: "This year's biggest cultural phenomenon in fashion can be seen on world-class athletes, presidential candidates, pop-culture icons and students all over campus . . . Lance Armstrong has the look everyone is going for" (1). Recently, I asked a close friend of mine where she got her bracelet. Her response: "My friend gave it to me." In this same article, McCoy interviews a freshman at the university named Trey Fletcher. His response was the same; the bracelet was given to him by a friend. If this holds true for many of the other teenagers wearing these bracelets, then it would appear as though the whole meaning behind them has been lost.

Wearing a Nike Livestrong bracelet is supposed to symbolize the fact that an individual spent one dollar to support the cure for cancer, but in many instances, people are not even directly purchasing the bracelet. Instead, these people rely on others to provide the bracelet to them. If people are relying on acquaintances to give them a bracelet, but not actually purchasing the product themselves, then why would one choose to wear the bracelet? The purpose behind the wristbands is to show society that you have done your role in supporting the cause for cancer by directly purchasing the product through the Lance Armstrong Foundation, and in effect, giving your own money to a possible cure. It seems as though once an individual feels that he/she can no longer "keep up with the Jones'," he will go to any extreme to fit in . . . even if it means falsely supporting a monumental issue such as cancer. For individuals like these, the bracelets act as a symbol of status and popularity, instead of a symbol for a possible cure for cancer. In any society, every individual is affected by advertising, and because of this effect on young adults and teenagers alike, the meaning behind these bracelets has been transformed.

It is sad that in the current age, individuals need to buy their way into acceptance. Many who yearn to be accepted by society purchase materials that resemble a sense of status. Jack Solomon, author of "Masters of Desire: The Culture of American Advertising," and co-editor of *Signs of Life in the USA: Readings on Popular Culture for Writers*, describes what a status symbol is, and more importantly, why individuals seek status symbols to increase their chances of being accepted by a certain group: "Status symbols, then, are signs that identify their possessors' place in social hierarchy, markers of rank and prestige. . . . Semiotically, what matters is the signal it sends, its value as a sign of power" (162). One may argue that these bracelets are only worth one dollar, so how can they act as a sign resembling one's great wealth and prestige? In this sense, the Livestrong bracelets, and those alike, are status symbols, not representing wealth, but status as a sign of physical and emotional power, strength, and richness of character. People such as Lance Armstrong, as well as Yuriy Borzakovsky, Hicham El Guerrouj, and Justin Gatlin are endorsers of the bracelet as well as visible proof that status can come in the form of personal strength, determination, and will-power. Many people look up to those Olympic athletes such as Borzakovsky, Guerrouj, and Gatlin all victors in the 2004 Olympics in the event of track and field. These three first-place winners in their event were wearing the bracelet when they crossed the finish line also. As a result, 300,000 bracelets were ordered the following day through the Lance Armstrong Foundation. This is proof that individuals seek this power and recognition that these athletes attain. The buyers of these bracelets did not all jump at once and say, let's buy one to support cancer. No, sadly they realized that these prevailing and physically powerful athletes wore one, so if they also wore one, they may be perceived the same (Layden 1).

Not only does Nike create bracelets that have transformed meaning, but Nike also produces a bracelet targeted to basketball players. This wristband guarantees false dignity and respect to all basketball players while on the court, something they cannot prove or support. The following is the advertisement for the Nike Baller ID Band which contains the unfulfilled guarantee by Nike to basketball players: "Recognized on the playground. Known in the gym. Respected for your game, your heart, your skill. Invited to every run. Welcome on any team. You're a baller"

(Lance Armstrong Foundation). Nike is promising teenagers who will buy into this deceptive ad, that if they wear this bracelet, their game will be respected, and they will be welcome to play anywhere exclusively because they are wearing the Baller ID Band. This is not the truth at all. Children who are not highly skilled at basketball cannot simply pick up a ball and think they can play with those who are at a much higher level, and also be respected for their skill level. This is the exact opposite of what will happen in a real-life situation. A basketball player may wear the bracelet with the mindset that everyone on the court will respect him or her regardless of the skill level they have, but we live in an extremely competitive world, especially when it comes to sports. In this sense Nike is making a promise to young kids and teenagers that they cannot truly fulfill. This is flat out false advertising. According to the *Merriam-Webster Dictionary of Law*, false advertising is, "the crime or tort of publishing, broadcasting, or otherwise publicly distributing an advertisement that contains an untrue, misleading, or deceptive representation or statement which was made knowingly or recklessly and with the intent to promote the sale of property, goods, or services to the public." This is exactly what Nike is doing with the Baller ID Band; they are publicly distributing an advertisement that may be misleading to young children and teenagers, selling this bracelet for a profit, knowing all along that they cannot promise the satisfaction they guarantee. The children and teenagers who buy into this deceptive ad truly believe that he or she will receive dignity and respect from others on the court, only because Nike is misleading these individuals to believe that it may be true. From the start, Lance Armstrong envisioned a product that was solely meant to raise money for a true cause. He never envisioned greedy businessmen using this idea to create a profit for themselves. Supporting the cause to raise money for cancer is a brilliant proposition, but companies should not capitalize on a product geared to raise money for this fatal disease which nearly 10 million people have today. Nike fed off of the reaction the consumers had with the popularity of the Livestrong bracelet and realized that many people would wear wristbands that resemble the Livestrong bracelet for the same reason the endorsers of the Livestrong bracelet are wearing them. This is immoral. Nike has used the Livestrong bracelet, something that began as a powerful cause, as a template, and capitalized on the bracelet by forming the Baller ID Band. In doing so, the inherent meaning behind the Livestrong bracelet was diminished because Nike adopted a new reasoning for the Baller ID Band. These new bracelets being produced are not going to a cause, rather they are solely manufactured to create business for themselves. Those who support the true cause behind the

Livestrong bracelets should recognize this and not be persuaded to buy the other bracelets Nike produces. Yet those who do purchase these spin-offs of the Livestrong bracelet are bandwagon consumers who have become sucked in by the appealing advertising proposed by greedy Nike marketers.

John De Graff, David Wann, and Thomas Naylor, all co-authors of an essay entitled "The Addictive Virus," all agree on one idea regarding consumerism in society today: consumers "are buying too much stuff, and all for the wrong reasons." The three later say that consumers are addicted to shopping because society forces individuals to shop for one reason; to increase one's self esteem. Many shop to be accepted, and as a result to increase their self esteem, and self-worth (De Graff et al. 71). Individuals are buying into the greedy and corrupt businessmen/woman who will go to any means to make money. Advertisers have used this flaw created by society, of which many consumers have. These selfish beings capitalized on these bracelets and turned them into something that people will want to buy to be accepted by society, instead of supporting the cure for cancer.

In his essay entitled, "The Spam Spoils of War," Damien Carve states his position regarding the capitalization of goods that should not be advertised, and the consumers who are affected by this capitalization. Carve is saying that manufacturers feed off of the emotions of consumers and use this as a means of making more money because the marketers know what the consumers want to buy (123). Nike saw that consumers everywhere lavished in the idea of the Livestrong bracelets, and as a result, thirty-one other versions of the bracelet have emerged. Some spin-offs such as the Muscular Dystrophy, Tobacco Free Kids, Aids, Support Our Troops, Ovarian Cancer and World Peace wristbands are following the same path as the Livestrong bracelets. Others such as "I Love My Cat," the "All in One" World Series bracelet, or the "Good Luck" band are being created for this very reason Carve explains in, "The Spam Spoils of War"; to make money (Livestrong). Their sole importance is to create more money for the company.

Selfishness is a quality that is inherently a part of all marketers who capitalize on the Livestrong bracelets, and it has sadly spread to ignorant consumers. Many individuals, not working for Nike or the Lance Armstrong Foundation, are selling bracelets for their own financial benefit. These bracelets cost one dollar through the Lance Armstrong foundation, but because they are in such demand, consumers will go to any means to purchase one. Because the bracelets have transformed into such a fashion trend, many will overlook the true support behind the bracelet, and possibly spend up to $20 for one on eBay, an online auction site. People who have Livestrong bracelets are selling them for much more than their actual price, only to gain a personal profit. None of the money produced by these bracelets on eBay is in fact going to the Lance Armstrong Foundation; it is rather going into the pockets of ignorant and selfish individuals who have the same mindset as corrupt marketers. Michelle Milford, a spokeswoman for the Lance Armstrong Foundation, was interviewed by Matt Hines, staff writer for CNET News. In his article entitled "Livestrong bands on eBay? It's not about charity," Michelle tells Matt the following regarding the selling of the Livestrong bracelets using eBay: "We're seeing them sold for as much as $20 in some cases, and we could put that money toward valuable research," Milford said. "The eBay situation is being caused by a perception that there is a shortage of bracelets, which there is not." Consumers are impatient. They cannot wait the two weeks for their bracelet to come in, so they resort to eBay to purchase one, sometimes for twenty times worth the actual value. This is proof that many are buying and wearing the bracelets for status, not to support cancer, and many individuals have turned into selfish marketers themselves by selling them via the internet and keeping this profit.

What will happen when people realize that marketers have overused this as an idea for an increase in business? People will stop wearing these bracelets, and the primary reason for these wristbands will be lost. The true reason behind the Livestrong bracelet will eventually lose its meaning because the capitalization on these bracelets by the marketer transformed their meaning from a sign of hope to a sign of public appeal and desire. Companies want us to believe that they are promoting their product for a significant reason, but in reality, their main objective is to make money.

In a consumer society, everything always comes back to the individual and what he or she can buy to become accepted or seem appealing by society. The focus of products changes from what the product is supposed to mean, to how the individual uses the product to make himself or herself more appealing to society, and also to create an identity for themselves. So long as a market exists, individuals will fall victim to it. The market cannot exist without these bandwagon consumers. With that said, is it simply inevitable that this vicious cycle will never end? For those of us who have been affected by cancer, directly or indirectly, and choose to support the cause by wearing the bracelet, this must be our only reasoning for wearing the Livestrong bracelet. We are right next to those who are fighting a long battle with cancer, those who are on the same road as Armstrong, as well as 10 million others worldwide. We will support them until they cross the finish line a victor. For those that wear this bracelet for the true meaning, I commend and support you. For those who wear it to increase your sense of appeal and to form your identity, I cannot wait for the day a bracelet is made stating, "Bandwagon Consumer," or, "Greedy Advertiser." If we as a society are going to wear our identity around our wrists, it might as well be truthful.

Works Cited

Capital Sports and Entertainment. "About Lance/Biography." Nov. 2004 <http://www.lancearmstrong.com/about.htm>.

Carve, Damien "The Spam Spoils of War" *Signs of Life in the USA: Readings on Popular Culture for Writers*. Ed. Sonia Maasik and Jack Solomon Boston: Bedford, St. Martin's, 2003.

Collector's Paradise. "Livestrong." Advertisement. Nov. 2004 <http://www.collectorsparadise.com/bracelets.html>.

De Graff, John, Wann, David, Naylor, Thomas H. "The Addictive Virus." *Signs of Life in the USA: Readings on Popular Culture for Writers*. Ed. Sonia Maasik and Jack Solomon Boston: Bedford, St. Martin's, 2003.

"False Advertising." *Merriam-Webster Dictionary of Law*. Nov. 2004 <http://dictionary.lp.findlaw.com>.

Hines, Matt "Livestrong Bands on eBay? It's not about Charity." <http://ecoustics-cnet.com>.

Lance Armstrong Foundation. "Livestrong Baller Id." Nov. 2004 Advertisement. <http://www.livestrongbracelets.net/>.

Layden, Tim. "Bracelet mania: Armstrong's Yellow Wrist Bands Have Become Cultural Phenomenon." *Sports Illustrated Magazine* 10 Sept. 2004

Solomon, Jack "Masters of Desire: The Culture of American Advertising" *Signs of Life in the USA: Readings on Popular Culture for Writers*. Ed. Sonia Maasik and Jack Solomon Boston, MA: Bedford, St. Martin's, 2003.

11   *Time to End the Epidemic*

Alyssa Somley

America's weight problem has become a national crisis. In the past few decades, Americans' lifestyles have shifted for the worse, creating an obesity epidemic. We are simply consuming too much food and not exercising enough. Obesity is defined as, "a condition characterized by excess body fat, typically defined in clinical settings as a body mass index (one's weight in kilograms divided by height in meters squared), of thirty or above" (Wardlaw 4). As it has recently become the second leading cause of preventable death in the United States, one would think that this dangerous increase in obesity would wake Americans up, but sadly it has not. Obesity is a serious issue that needs to be dealt with, causing serious health risks like heart disease, high blood pressure, stroke, diabetes, infertility, gallbladder disease, osteoarthritis and many forms of cancer. The epidemic has become real and because our collective health has been getting progressively worse, today's kids may be the first generation in history whose life expectancy is projected to be less than that of their parents (Lemonick and Bjerklie 60).

Unfortunately, with the growing access to fast food and advancements in transportation technology, it does not look like Americans are going to start changing their lifestyles anytime soon. The media has recognized the trouble America is in, and has decided to try to help. They use shocking, unappealing images when discussing obesity to attempt to educate Americans, in hopes that they will change their ways. The methods used to depict obesity in the media are diverse, each source taking a different approach when dealing with the issue; however they all work towards making Americans aware of the seriousness of the rising obesity epidemic. *Time* magazine has become a major player in alerting Americans to the crisis we have on our hands. As a popular magazine, *Time* educates its readers about the seriousness of obesity, and as the issue has evolved over time, *Time* has evolved as well, targeting the average American in hopes that it can make a difference.

In June of 2004, Michael Lemonick and David Bjerklie of *Time* wrote an article called "How We Grew So BIG." This article argues that poor diet and lack of exercise are immediate causes of obesity, but our problem is a result of our transforming environment. Lemonick and Bjerklie support their article by stating:

> Although our physiology has stayed pretty much the same for the past 50,000 years or so, we humans have utterly transformed our environment. Over the past century, especially, technology has almost completely removed physical exercise from the day-to-day lives of most Americans. At the same time, it has filled supermarket shelves with cheap, mass-produced, good-tasting food that is packed with calories. And finally, technology has allowed advertisers to deliver constant, virtually irresistible messages that say "Eat this now" to everyone old enough to watch TV. (58)

This simple argument helps the reader to understand how our transforming environment has contributed to this obesity problem.

Lemonick and Bjerklie's article does a great job covering obesity in general. It addresses the rising epidemic with statistics such as:

> Fully two-thirds of U.S. adults are officially overweight, and about half of those have graduated to full-blown obesity. The rates for African Americans and Latinos are even higher. Among kids between 6 and 19 years old, 15%, or 1 in 6, are overweight, and another 15% are headed that way. Even our pets are pudgy: a depressing 25% of dogs and cats are heavier than they should be. (58)

By providing a background of what obesity is, the seriousness of it, and why it is rising, the article is setting the tone for its readers. It is educating this average American reader to help them become aware of the issue.

The topic of obesity continues to evolve every day. Time continues to cover the epidemic in hopes that it can further educate its readers by producing articles that are more and more focused on the dangerous symptoms of obesity. Six months after "How We Grew So BIG," Jeffrey Kluger of *Time* wrote an article called, "Blowing a Gasket." This article is specifically focused on the fluctuation of high blood pressure in Americans, which is ultimately caused by obesity.

"At least 65 million Americans—a third of all adults over 18—are thought to suffer from hypertension (the technical term for persistent high blood pressure), up from 50 million just 10 years ago" (Kluger 74). This statistic mirrors the studies done on obesity. The bottom line is that as obesity is increasing, its symptoms are fluctuating as well. Instead of focusing on the broad subject of obesity, Time is now focusing in on specific symptoms Americans should know about so that they can slowly resolve each one, ultimately leading to a healthier lifestyle and a stop to the epidemic.

"Blowing a Gasket" goes on to discuss the rise in hypertension now being seen in kids as they too are becoming increasingly overweight. With the help of pictures and diagrams, the article makes it easy for the average reader to understand the complicated issue. Like "How We Grew So BIG," it gives background information on the topic as well as ways we can fight this increase in hypertension. No matter how many other factors may contribute to hypertension, the article continues to emphasize its point that the number one reason Americans are suffering from high blood pressure is due to obesity. "Worse, the 65 million figure is just an estimate of the vulnerable population, and that population is a constantly moving target. Every time the nation's obesity needle ticks upward, the number of hypertensive Americans does too" (Kluger 78). And so, as the issue of obesity has evolved, so has Time, converting to discussing symptoms of obesity in hopes that it can fight the epidemic one step at a time.

"How We Grew So BIG," was the perfect article for Time to begin to educate their readers about America's rising obesity problem. The statistics and reasoning behind the epidemic were simple and geared towards the average reader. This technique made the article very persuasive because the readers could relate to and understand the information. While trying to explain to its readers why the obesity epidemic is a result of our evolving environment, Lemonick and Bjerklie make a simple point:

> And thanks to mass production, all that food is relatively cheap. It's also absurdly convenient. In many areas of the U.S., if you had a craving for cookies a century ago, you had to fire up the woodstove and make the dough from scratch. If you wanted butter, you had to churn it. If you wanted a steak, you had to butcher the cow. Now you jump into the car and head for the nearest convenience store or if that's too much effort, you pick up a phone or log on to the Internet and have the stuff delivered to your door. (60)

This argument is obvious and makes sense, thus creating a sense of confidence and ultimately persuading the reader.

For the average American reader, I feel that *Time* is a trustworthy source. It provides honest information, but in a way that interests the readers. For example, Lemonick and Bjerklie make this statistic stand out on the first page of the article:

> Twenty years ago, 5% of American kids were overweight; today 15% are, and another 15% are headed that way. In 1969 80% of kids played sports every day; today 20% do. By 17, a child has spent 38% more time in front of the TV than in school. (59)

Time realizes that the people who are going to buy their magazine are most likely adults because they are the ones who do the shopping and have the money. Most adults today have children, and so *Time* uses statistics like the one above to draw their attention and make them want to read on. The statistics are true, the information is valid, and they relate to their largest audience. Although *Time* may not choose to use the most scientific information, due to the fact that their articles must be interesting to make a profit, the information they do use is valid. However, if you were a professional, someone specialized on the subject, looking for up to date information, you would not refer to *Time*. An academic journal like *JAMA* (the *Journal of the American Medical Association*), would be more appropriate because it is geared towards educating the willing and does not need to use flashy pictures and statistics to appeal to its reader. Instead, it uses scientifically proven statistics and information that have gone through a rigorous testing process by professionals to make sure the information is accurate.

The use of images also contributes to *Time*'s arguments. On the cover of "How We Grew So BIG," is an obese white male, standing at the end of an almost broken diving board, while his overweight family watches on, laughing at this incredible sight. From the children to the dog, the whole family is clearly overweight. The large portions of food sitting in the background along with the lack of activity shown is *Time*'s way of explaining why Americans become obese. Although this image may not be a correct portrayal of the "average obese family," this is an example of the types of images popular magazines will use to evoke feelings and interest in the average American. I feel *Time* is using this unappealing image to accompany the article to try to scare their viewers and help make them aware of the problem our society has.

Time, like every other source in the media is ultimately working towards one goal: to make Americans aware of the seriousness of the obesity epidemic. "How We Grew So BIG," did an excellent job of stressing the seriousness of the problem. With the use of flashy pictures, like the unappealing obese family on the cover page, it created a sense of shock in the reader. Lemonick and Bjerklie also stressed statistics like, "Just two decades ago, the incidence of overweight in adults was well under 50%, while the rate for kids was only one third what it is today. From 1996 to 2001, two million teenagers and young adults joined the ranks of the clinically obese" (58). Statistics like this reach out to the average reader and make them further aware of America's obesity problem. The article was very persuasive because it was based on a simple argument that made sense: that diet and lack of exercise are immediate causes of obesity, but our problem is a result of our transforming environment. *Time's* articles are doing a great job of helping make Americans aware of the problem we have on our hands. It appeals to a large portion of the American population, and continues to evolve and educate readers as the issue of obesity evolves. Hopefully, this new technique of focusing in on specific symptoms of obesity will help tackle the epidemic one step, and one reader, at a time.

Works Cited

Kluger, Jeffrey. "Blowing a Gasket." *Time* 6 Dec. 2004: 73-80.

Lemonick, Michael, and David Bjerklie. "How We Grew So BIG." *Time* 7 June 2004: 58-65.

Wardlaw, Gordon M. *Contemporary Nutrition: Issues and Insights*. 5th ed. Boston: McGraw Hill, 2003.

The
Persuasive Researched
Essay

12 Whose Fault Is it Anyway?

Brad Solomon

My cousin and I have smoked cigarettes since right around the time we started selling cars. At first, we went through the quintessential "OPC" (other peoples' cigarettes) stage, in which we strategically waited for one of our smoking coworkers to walk out the back door. One of us would always walk out first and ask, "Hey do you have an extra by any chance," while the other sat inside. After about forty-five seconds, whichever of us was still butt-less would walk out of the building and, of course, say the same thing. It became a joke around the dealership; we were the "one-two punch." As is generally the case, though, Matt and I soon began looking at cigarettes not as something to pass the time, but as a stress reliever, a way to calm down. When we began buying packs, we admitted to ourselves that we were now smokers; the addiction process had run its course.

So as I sit here, staring at my depressingly empty pack of Marlboro Lights, I ask myself, "How the hell did this happen?" I used to be a big, weight-lifting, protein shake-drinking health nut that wouldn't even eat fried chicken. Now, I can't fathom the thought of walking to or from class without smoking a cigarette. Do I feel ashamed? No, because I like smoking cigarettes. Do I feel victimized? No, because I made my own decision to start. I knew what I was doing when I lit that first cigarette, and I will accept the consequences for my choice. I'm not interested in examining only my personal situation, though. I'm looking at this on a much broader basis. What factors lead a society to participate in such a disgusting habit on such a large scale? Who and what are the real influences that cause so many to participate in the leading cause of preventable death in the United States?

Many people believe that tobacco advertising is the sole reason Americans are so addicted to cigarettes. Indeed, studies have shown that tobacco companies successfully promote their products by using attractive models, attractive lifestyles, and attractive feelings. It has also been proven that tobacco companies heavily target America's youth, as this age demographic is most susceptible to cigarette addiction. In fact, if one does not become a smoker before he turns 18 years old, he is ninety percent less likely to become a smoker later in life. By primarily advertising toward youth, tobacco companies have certainly made a significant contribution to the problem ("FDA Justified").

Quite frankly, though, I'm tired of advertisers singlehandedly absorbing the punishment for society's sins simply. There are many ignored factors that play into America's addiction to tobacco, and we can't place all responsibility for America's tobacco problems in the hands of the advertising industry. The problem is too serious for one group of professionals to take all the blame. State governments, the Federal government, Hollywood, and even parents have unconsciously fostered the development of the tobacco industry, with no help from the industry itself. Americans have allowed for, and knowingly contributed to, the creation of a society that openly accepts smoking.

The Ad Man

Am I absolving advertisers of all blame? Certainly not. I stated earlier that it has been proven that advertisers target children in order to hook new smokers when they are not mentally ready to make an intelligent decision. Furthermore, if cigarette manufacturers decided to discontinue all cigarettes, the problem would clear up pretty quickly. The product they manufacture kills 440,000 people per year. Luckily for them, though, 1.63 million non-smokers (757,000 of whom are under age eighteen) convince themselves to join the fun each year ("Trends in Tobacco").

Let it be known, though, that tobacco advertisers have had some pretty heavy restrictions put on them. In 1998, the Master Settlement Agreement, in which forty-six states sued the four largest tobacco companies for billions of dollars in health care losses, called for numerous changes in tobacco advertising laws. While it has been a long time since tobacco companies have been allowed to run TV ads, 1998's agreement stripped the companies of their right to advertise on billboards. Also, the MSA called for the removal of all youth targeted advertising, including the complete demise of one Joe Camel. Tobacco companies are also not allowed to advertise in magazines "with more than 2 million readers younger than 18 or with more than 15 percent youth readership" ("Tobacco Companies Target").

The MSA did not completely stop the tobacco industry from marketing to minors, though. In fact, tobacco companies have recently been scrutinized for specifically targeting the youth in certain minority groups. RJ Reynolds, maker of Kool and Camel cigarettes, was recently accused of "using hip-hop images to seduce minority youth into smoking." This accusation was the result of Kool's production of Smooth Fusion, Mixx, and Camel Exotic Blends. Sherri Watson Hyde, executive director of the National African American Tobacco Prevention Network, argues, "What adult that you know prefers a tropical or berry-flavored cigarette?" ("Hip-Hop Images").

Other youth-targeted advertising methods have recently been examined, including convenience stores' placement of cigarette signs at a child's eye level. Also, tobacco companies have found, and capitalized on, a loophole in 1998's Master Settlement Agreement. As previously stated, the Agreement stated that tobacco companies may not advertise in magazines "with more than 2 million readers younger than 18 or with more than 15 percent youth readership." However, a study in Nation's Health magazine found that after this restriction was put on them, "tobacco companies began concentrating their advertising to magazines that fell just below the FDA limits when compared to their advertising efforts before the multistate agreement. The closer readership was to the FDA levels, the more likely the tobacco companies focused on those magazines" ("Tobacco Companies Target").

The State Blunder

So, I acknowledge that advertisers certainly do contribute to America's smoking problem. As previously stated, though, my goal for this essay is to expose many contributing factors that have gone unnoticed. For example, it seems dishonorable for the tobacco companies to come so close to the magazine advertising limits in the Master Settlement Agreement. However, let us not forget that this document was drawn up by forty-six individual state governments ("FDA Justified"). These elected officials were experienced, intelligent, and hopefully had in mind the best interest of their citizens. Why, then, couldn't they think of a more innovative way compose the Agreement such that tobacco companies weren't able to find such an obvious loophole? I'll give the states the benefit of the doubt, and assume this was a blunder. Perhaps they should have spent more time discussing and rewriting the Agreement. What if it wasn't a blunder, though? It should be known that the state governments collect 20 billion dollars annually from "sin taxes" on cigarettes. Am I supposed to trust my elected officials when they say they're fighting against America's tobacco problem? In reality, states allocate approximately 538 million dollars annually to tobacco prevention, a figure that equals one-third of the Centers for Disease Control and Prevention (CDC) suggested funds allocation. In this instance, the individual state governments have either directly or indirectly contributed to this country's smoking problem without accepting any of the responsibility.

TRUTH or DARE

The individual state governments aren't the only governments responsible for America's smoking problem. The federal government has played a part by continuing funding for DARE (Drug Abuse Resistance Education) and ignoring the tobacco prevention program TRUTH. DARE is designed to make elementary school children aware of the dangers of tobacco and other drugs. Of course, I'm not attacking the underlying concept behind DARE. However, it has been proven that the program in extremely ineffective; it is a waste of 750 million dollars annually, and is an example of the federal government's fiscal irresponsibility (West). Not surprisingly, there have been no studies in the program's eighteen-year history indicating its effectiveness, but there have been numerous studies indicating its ineffectiveness (Szalavitz). In the words of Kathy Stewart, resident of the UTAH DARE Officer's Association, "I don't have any statistics for you. Our strongest numbers are the numbers that don't show up" (Sullum). On the other hand, TRUTH is the most successful anti-smoking campaign ever created. In the two years following its debut, 1 million high school smokers kicked the habit, representing a five percent decrease. The program has been funded by a portion of the money awarded to the individual states as a result of the 1998 Master Settlement Agreement. Now, though, TRUTH's funding is in danger of being cut because states have been using the rest of this money for causes other than tobacco prevention (Krisberg). If TRUTH does lose its funding and is forced to dissolve, the only advocacy for tobacco prevention in this country will be in the hands of DARE and the tobacco companies. If the federal government wishes to lessen America's smoking problem instead of further contributing to it, it will cut DARE funding and send more monies in the way of TRUTH. Otherwise, Americans' tax dollars will continue to go to waste, and the tobacco problem will not improve.

Hollywood Smoke

OK, "Big deal," you might be saying. I've managed to point out the ways in which our politicians screw things up. How original, right? For those of you who are wondering if there's any real merit to my argument, let's switch gears and examine the behaviors of some truly admired members of our society.

A 2003 survey conducted by researchers at Dartmouth Medical School concluded that "watching popular movies is the No. 1 factor leading non-smoking teens to light up. Smoking in movies is having a major effect on [public] health." (Batchelor). These findings make perfect sense; people emulate the trends presented in popular movies. For proof of this sentiment, look no further than 1983's *Risky Business*. When Tom Cruise danced around in his underwear while wearing Ray Ban Wayfarer sunglasses, the sunglasses suddenly became "chic," and "within weeks of [the movie's] release, the $55-a-pair ebony Wayfarers were walking off the shelves" (Pouschine). Look, also, at the childish nostalgia generated by 2004's Ben Stiller hit, *Dodgeball*. Since the movie's release, *Dodgeball* leagues have been popping up in locations all over North America; teams such as "The Bling" and the "Beef Sharks" can be seen on Game Show Network's *Extreme Dodgeball* every Thursday at 10 PM et. (Deziel).

Now that the correlation between movie behavior and real-life behavior has been established, I will assume the Dartmouth study was at least partially accurate. Should I point the cigarette finger at Baz Luhrmann, who directed 1996's *Romeo & Juliet*, in which Leonardo DiCaprio is shown smoking (Distefan)? To his credit, I'm sure Luhrmann felt strongly that the cigarette was important to the progression of the movie. However, since he was releasing a PG-13 movie targeted at young adults, should his ethics have taken precedence over his artistic sense? For that matter, should I even let DiCaprio off the hook? If I remember correctly, DiCaprio was 1996's equivalent to 1983's Tom Cruise, quite an influential icon. As a matter of fact, I remember two things about my life when this movie came out: 1) I couldn't get any girls to like me because 2) they were all gaga over Leonardo DiCaprio. I'm not implying that DiCaprio or Luhrmann were paid to incorporate cigarettes in this movie, but they should use better judgement when choosing a movie's props.

Sharon Stone is another big-name star who has unintentionally contributed to America's tobacco problem. Ironically enough, she was at UNH during John Kerry's campaign, advocating stem cell research. When I left her speech, I said to myself, "Hey, I like her cause." Then I realized that she smokes in *Casino*, as well as in many other movies. Sure, *Casino* is an R-rated movie, so any teenager who sees the movie is doing so illegally. Did this stop any of us in high school, though? I know *Casino* was the movie of choice in my school. If Stone is going to advocate for stem cell research, she really should have thought twice about lighting up in this movie. Perhaps if less adolescents started smoking, stem cell research would be less of a necessity.

While on the subject of movies, I'd like to have a round-table discussion with Kevin J. Martin, chairman of the FCC, and Dan Glickman, President of the Motion Picture Association of America. I'd like to discuss with these two men the inadequacies and hypocrisies associated with smoking in films. Interestingly enough, a movie gets an R rating if the "F-word" is used more than once, or only once in a "sexual context" (Batchelor). Smoking has seemingly been overlooked, though. So, Kevin and Dan, it's okay if people are contracting emphysema and lung cancer, as long as they're not swearing in the hospital bed, right?

Tube-acco

Following my research of the motion picture industry's effect on adolescent smoking, I felt it also would be necessary to examine television's influence on the problem. I assumed there had to be a significant correlation, as it is common knowledge that people are influenced by what they see on TV. As it turns out, I was right. Children and adolescents that view actors smoking on television are more likely to become smokers. Programs such as Seinfeld, music videos, and many medical dramas are believed to present a substantial amount of glorified smoking. More importantly, though, the content children watch is less influential than the sheer amount of time they spend watching anything. Furthermore, there is an "upsloping" relationship between the amount of TV adolescents watch and the amount of cigarettes they smoke (Gutschoven). A reasonable explanation for this is that "children learn to associate TV viewing with eating, snacking, or drinking early on, for instance, because they are breast- or bottle-fed while their parents watch TV. In a similar vein, children might learn to see smoking as something which is a normal thing to do when watching the television" (Gutschoven).

Mom's Role

The information regarding the relationship between television and smoking is disturbing, because it's unclear on whom society should place the blame. Can we blame the television industry itself? Yes, because TV shows do show smoking in a positive light, which influences people to mimic the behavior. However, since content is less important than time spent, America's parents must be held largely accountable for adolescent smoking. The following statistics, produced by the A.C. Nielsen Company, illustrate the television habits our society has developed:

Number of hours per day the television is on in an average U.S. home: 6 hours, 47 minutes. Number of minutes per week that the average child watches television: 1,680. Hours per year the average American youth watches television: 1,500. ("TV Stats")

In lieu of these findings, is it too bold an assertion to say that America's parents must be held at least partially accountable for adolescent smoking? Presumably, parents hold the authority to set limits on the amount of time their children spend in front of the tube, so it is parents' fault that the average child endures so much overexposure. Therefore, since TV viewing is directly related to smoking, America's smoking problem actually starts in the home, on the couch, while Mom and Dad are at work. Interesting . . . who would have thought that a generation of children raised by a television instead of their own parents would take solace in smoking cigarettes? It's pretty safe to say that many of these young TV addicts find cigarettes an acceptable manner of attracting much-needed attention.

Conclusion

It can be argued that advertisers are mostly responsible for tobacco's prevalence on a large scale. But on a small, one-person scale, I believe we are all responsible for examining all of our actions and their effects on the rest of the world. At the beginning of this assignment, I just wanted to answer one question for myself: would I work for Phillip Morris? I now know the truth, that I already work for Phillip Morris, and didn't even know it. Every time I'm seen lighting a cigarette, I am a walking advertisement. Every time I rent a movie that contains a smoking scene, I contribute to the problem; I should be boycotting the movie and writing letters to the producers. Every time I give a cigarette to a friend, girlfriend, or random kid at a party, I am promoting cigarette use. Now that I think about it, my cousin might live a shorter life because of me. If more organizations could come to this same realization, that their actions affect people in ways of which they aren't even aware, huge improvements would be made against America's smoking problem.

Works Cited

Batchelor, Suzanne. "Movie Smoking Hooks Teens, Experts Say." *National Catholic Reporter*. 6 February 2004.

Centers for Disease Control and Prevention. <www.cdc.gov>.

Deziel, Shanda. "Unartful dodgers of adulthood." *Maclean's*. 14 March 2005. 118 (11).

Distefan, Janet M., John P. Pierce, Elizabeth A. Gilpin. "Do Favorite Movie Stars Influence Adolescent Smoking Initiation?" *American Journal of Public Health*. July 2004: 94 (7).

"FDA Justified in Regulating Tobacco Advertising Targeting Youth" *The Brown University Digest of Addiction Theory & Application*. June 1997: 16 (6).

Gutschoven, Klass and Jan Van den Bulck. "Television viewing and smoking volume in adolescent smokers: a cross-sectional study." *Preventive Medicine*. 7 June 2004. 39.

Heil, Emily. ". . . As Foes Caution about Slippery Slope of Regulations." *CongressDaily*. 11 August 2004.

Henriksen, Lisa, Ellen C. Feighery, Yun Wang, Stephen P. Fortmann. "Association of Retail Tobacco Marketing With Adolescent Smoking." *American Journal of Public Health*. December 2004: 94 (12).

"Hip-Hop Images Blamed for Seducing Minority Youth Into Smoking." *Black Issues in Higher Education*. 9 September 2004. 21 (15).

Krisberg, Kim. "Successful 'truth' anti-smoking campaign in funding jeopardy." *Nation's Health*. May 2004: 34 (4).

National Center for Policy Analysis. http://www.ncpa.org/pi/taxes/ tax41.html.

Pouschine, Tatiana. "Cruising on Ray-Bans." *Forbes*. 3 August 1992. 150 (3).

Shadel, William G., Raymond Niaura, David B. Abrams. "Adolescents' responses to the gender valence of cigarette advertising imagery: The role of affect and the self-concept." Department of Psychology, University of Pittsburgh.

Sullum, Jacob. "DARE AWARE." *Reason*. Jan. 2001. 32 (8).

Szalavitz, Maia. "Dare to Change." *New Scientist*. Feb. 2002. 173 (2328).

"Television Statistics." *TV-Free America*. <http://www.csun.edu/ ~vceed002/health/docs/tv&health.html>.

"Tobacco Companies Continue to Target Teens Through Ads." *Nation's Health*. May 2002: 32 (4).

"Trends in Tobacco Use." *American Lung Association.* <http://www.lungusa.org/atf/cf/{7A8D42C2-FCCA-4604-8ADE-7F5D5E762256}/SMK1.PDF>.

West, Steven L. and Keri K. O'Neal. "Project D.A.R.E. Outcome Effectiveness Revisited." *American Journal of Public Health.* June 2004: 94 (6).

13

The Ideals of Amateurism vs. the Reality of Sport: Should Division I College Athletes be Paid?

Dan Jasinski

Sports have long held a prominence in American culture, more so than in most other places of the world. There are entire television networks dedicated solely to the covering of the world of sports, and one would have a hard time finding a person who has never read the sports page of their local newspaper. In any athletic competition, a team sport or an individual event, many of the ideals that make up the fabric of American culture are easily visible. The importance of working together for a common goal, the need to sacrifice oneself for the greater good, the necessity of determination and perseverance, all of these aspects are on display during athletic competition. This is especially true in amateur athletics, where without the influence of money, competitors play simply for "the love of the game." However, when one looks at the world of college sports, especially the larger sports such as football and basketball, it becomes necessary to examine what exactly constitutes an amateur athlete. Gone are the idyllic days of athletes in these sports playing solely for the pride of their school; in its place are million-dollar bowl games, billion-dollar television contracts and illegal payments from program boosters looking to help their favorite player. After examining the world of college sports and determining where the money from athletic events flows, it seems clear that a change is necessary within the National Collegiate Athletic Association (NCAA) rules regarding player compensation. In order to fairly balance the importance of amateurism in college athletics while still accepting the reality of the world of college sports, the NCAA should modify its rules to allow athletes to accept endorsements for their athletic ability while in college. These changes would need to be monitored closely, however provided that they were, these rules would allow athletes to be fairly rewarded for their efforts while still promoting the values of amateurism and the meaning of the student athlete.

The Money Trail

It is at best naïve to deny that NCAA Division I football and basketball have turned into, or at least created multimillion-dollar industries. Every March, people in offices around the country gather together to fill out their brackets; that is to say that they make their predictions for the outcome of the annual NCAA men's basketball tournament, nicknamed "March Madness." As the opening rounds begin, millions settle into their couches and tune into CBS to watch the action unfold. The reason that all eyes are on CBS is because that is the network that won the bidding war when the contract for the rights to broadcast the games went up for sale in 1999. In exchange for the rights to broadcast the men's tournament for eleven years, CBS agreed to pay the NCAA 6 billion dollars. Every year, that money is distributed among the member institutions of the NCAA, who in turn use it to fund athletic teams at their respective schools. In addition, according to Kelly Whiteside of *USA Today*, the twenty-eight postseason bowls that are played every winter in football bring in a total of 184 million dollars, which is redistributed among the Division I football conferences (Whiteside par. 1).

This does not include money that is generated through corporate sponsorship of the NCAA's eighty-seven championship games. Darren Rovell of ESPN.com notes that "Under the NCAA Corporate Partner Program, 16 companies with household names such as Pepsi, General Motors and Sears Roebuck & Co., pay between 1.8 million dollars and 4 million dollars annually to associate their brands with 87 championship tournaments" (par. 3). Add on to this the revenue generated from merchandise sales at the different schools, and it is clear that there is an abundance of money being made off of what is supposed to be amateur athletic competition. It seems rather hypocritical to promote the notion of amateurism while then allowing these same amateurs to compete in the Continental Tire Bowl, the Big XII Championship presented by Dr. Pepper, or the FedEx Orange Bowl.

It becomes necessary to determine where the money that is clearly being made off of college football and basketball is going. Of the 370 million dollars that the NCAA received as a result of the basketball contract with CBS, approximately 253 million dollars went on to the various conferences and schools that comprise the NCAA (Suggs par. 14). The amount of money that is distributed to each conference or institution depends on a variety of factors, but includes how well conference teams have played in the basketball tournament in the past, how many sports the school sponsors, and how many scholarships the school grants to athletes (Suggs par. 16). This leads to a disparity in revenue flow as the larger, more skilled conferences and schools are in line to receive much more money than smaller conferences and schools. One can see this by noting the disparity in revenue between the conferences with major football and basketball programs, and those that compete on a smaller scale. In 2002–2003, the Southeastern Conference reported revenues of 122 million dollars, the most of any NCAA conference, while the Northeast Conference reported revenues of slightly over 1 million dollars (Suggs par. 34). Again, when speaking on conferences and schools with large-scale football and basketball programs, it is clear that there is a large amount of money being made off of what is supposed to be amateur competitions.

Once this money reaches the schools, it is first used to cover the funds for the athletic department, which is responsible for maintaining all of the athletic teams of the school. For example, the Ohio State University athletic department reported revenues of 50 million dollars in 2000, which covered all 37 varsity sports and netted the athletic department a profit of 3.51 million dollars (Glasser par. 2). Since athletic director Andy Geiger arrived at OSU in 1992, the school has spent 331.7 million dollars on athletic facilities, the money coming from public taxes, alumni and the school itself (Glassner par. 1). This is an enormous sum of money that has been spent on athletes that are supposed to be amateurs. That is not to say that amateurs deserve poor facilities, or that money should not be spent on college sports. However, author Jeff Glasser does an excellent job of noting exactly what this amount of money represents. He notes on page 5 that "Put another way, the university has spent $351,111.11 per varsity athlete on sports facilities, compared with $6,652 per student on other university buildings." This demonstrates the fact that, if athletics are not the top priority at Ohio State, they have at least been brought to the forefront in recent years.

Applied to a more broad level, this number can be compared to the estimated 395 million dollars that the Arizona Cardinals of the National Football League expect to pay for a new stadium, according to a report published by a finance committee from the San Diego city government (Horrow par. 1). When colleges are allowed to spend money that is close to, and in some cases more than, what professional teams spend on their facilities, what does that say about the people who are using the facilities? Professional teams build elite facilities for the purpose of attracting elite athletes in order to make money. The most recent stadium expansion at Ohio State brought the capacity of the stadium to 102,000 (Glasser par. 5). This is larger than any professional football stadium currently in use. When college athletes are given comparable facilities to professional athletes, use resources that are as good as, if not better than, their professional counterparts and bring more people to the games than the professionals, how can one say that there is much of a difference between the two.

Full-Time Job?

Beyond the similarity in facilities and resources, the schedule of a college athlete is similar to that of professional athletes as well. In an interview that I conducted with University of New Hampshire freshman Mike Radja, a member of the men's ice hockey team, he stated that the hockey team practices every day during the season for two hours in the afternoon, with off-ice conditioning two days a week in the morning. The hockey team plays around forty games per year, with approximately half being on the road, meaning that travel on the weekends is necessary on more than a few occasions. Furthermore, during the off season, the team meets every day of the week except for Sunday to work on conditioning. This is all done in addition to taking a normal class load, and the homework and preparation that goes along with being a regular student. This schedule bears more resemblance to those of a professional athlete than a typical college student. However, unlike the professional who only has to focus on his athletics, these student athletes have to make sure that their grades meet NCAA standards so that they maintain their eligibility. When these student athletes are spending well over twenty hours per week training and practicing for their sport, it seems clear that they deserve the opportunity for some type of reward for their effort. This is especially true in cases involving schools with prominent football or basketball teams, as these athletes often come from lower income families. What develops is a situation where the athlete feels that they are the people putting in the effort at practices and games, bringing the television contracts and notoriety to the NCAA and their school. They also see that they are the only ones who do not appear to be cashing in off the product that they are creating. The desire for money, even if it is just a few dollars to spend at the mall, is what causes many players to seek out the boosters that will give an athlete an illegal payment. However, if the NCAA were to give an outlet to this desire by changing their rules to allow players to earn outside compensation for their athletic abilities, players would have an opportunity to earn money because of their efforts while still keeping their eligibility.

College is not for Professionals

Those who are against allowing college athletes to be paid have two main arguments, both of which raise valid issues. The first argument is that the athletes already receive compensation, which takes the form of either a full or partial athletic scholarship. During the interview with Radja, he noted that in addition to receiving some type of scholarship, the equipment that the players use is provided to them free of charge. At UNH, with out of state tuition at almost $27,000, after adding in the cost of equipment one could argue that hockey players receive an annual salary of approximately $30,000. Over a typical four-year college stay, this amounts to around $120,000 in financial aid given to an out of state athlete, which is by no means a small sum of money. During our interview, Radja noted that "Most athletes are on some sort of scholarship, whether it is full or partial. There is a lot of money being invested in each athlete to perform, so the way I look at it its almost like getting paid."

It is important to note what kinds of restrictions are placed on an athlete when they receive an athletic scholarship. For example, a student who is on a scholarship for academic abilities must obviously keep their grade point average at a certain level, just as the athlete must earn at least a minimum of twelve credit hours per semester as defined by the NCAA rules regarding player eligibility (*NCAA Manual* 132). The student on an academic scholarship has some flexibility regarding their schedule and, should they desire, have time to work a part-time job. However, for athletes at the upper level of Division I competition, this is simply not an option. Furthermore, as stated on page 77-78 of the NCAA Division I Manual, athletes are not permitted to use their face or likeness to promote any sport specific instruction they may be offering, and are not allowed to offer playing lessons pertaining to their sport. Yet the student who is on the academic scholarship may be a tutor in his or her specialty, thereby making money off of his or her individual skills. Again, it seems hypocritical that the NCAA, in its efforts to promote the values of the student athlete, would not allow an athlete to support themselves in a way that is similar to that of a regular student.

The second argument that those who are against the payment of college athletes point to is a more ideological claim regarding the amateur nature of college sports. I do not dispute the argument that part of the reason that college sports are so special is because of the fact that, at least on the surface, there is no money involved for the player. This creates an environment of pure sport, one that is lacking in today's world of exorbitant professional salaries and labor disputes. There is something that is unique about college sports that is due to the relationship between athletes, students, and the community that they live in. When asked about this relationship, Mike Radja noted that "I haven't had any problems with students that weren't athletes," and that "as an athlete if we got paid it would be unreal, but I would be a little bitter if I was just another student." Clearly, the image of a sporting environment comprised entirely of amateurs and the aura that comes with it would be lost if athletes were paid.

However, if one takes an honest look at the world of college sports, one will surely notice that this world of amateur sports is not nearly as pure as we would like to believe. Andrew Stein states in an article for CNNMoney.com that since the mid-1970s, Nike and other shoe companies have been in a bidding war amongst the upper echelon of basketball schools for contracts with the school to wear their products. The wars started with paying coaches to ensure that their players wore a certain company's shoe, then moved on to signing contracts with the entire school to license all school merchandise (Stein par. 1). Furthermore, it seems that every year on the news there are stories like that of Troy Smith, a quarterback at Ohio State. Smith was suspended from his team's bowl game as a punishment for taking payments from a football booster, and will have to apply for reinstatement to the team over the off-season (ESPN.com par. 3). This is far from an isolated incident, and a brief check of sports pages will reveal that these acts occur with shocking regularity. Therefore, it seems those who point to Division I college athletics as being a beacon for the purity of amateur sport are naïve to the reality of what major college athletics has become.

Reconciling Reality and Ideals

Since all of the issues regarding player compensation have been exposed, the question now involves creating a system that attempts to balance all of the conflicting views. It would be far too cynical to say that college athletes are the same as professional athletes, yet naïve to say that they are all pure amateurs. Therefore, it would make sense to propose a change in the NCAA rules regarding player compensation that would allow a player to accept some kind of compensation for their athletic ability that was not like the regular salary that a professional would receive.

The first step to creating this system is to determine where the money for paying the athletes would come from. While there athletic departments that do bring in a profit, Whiteside notes that only forty of the nearly 1,000 member schools of the NCAA reported a profit (Whiteside par. 1). However, Goff notes in his study that these numbers are often construed to make the situation seem worse than it actually is. Schools can report money in ways that make it seem as though the source was not athletics, or can defer funds brought in by athletics to other departments and not note the move. After adding in revenue brought in by athlete tuition, and lowering the grant that the NCAA gives to schools based on the amount of athletes they house to accurately reflect what it costs the school to house athletes, Goff figured that the Utah State athletic department was off on their estimated revenue. Their numbers, published in 1988, showed a loss of $680,000; after Goff's calculations, they showed a gain of $360,000 (par. 4). Even though many schools could afford to pay their athletes some kind of stipend, this would not be in accordance with the goal of not giving athletes a regular salary, and would certainly put a strain on student-athlete relations if the regular student population felt that athletes were getting even more money from the school. In addition, schools that do not participate in the revenue attracting sports would not have the extra funds available to pay their athletes. However, there is another alternative that would allow athletes to receive some compensation for their efforts without giving them a regular salary and without costing the schools a penny.

The solution to this problem lies in the corporate sponsors of the NCAA. Currently, companies such as Nike, Bauer, Reebok, and numerous other athletic wear manufacturers have contracts with schools to outfit their teams and school merchandise. Every time a team with Nike shoes goes far into the NCAA basketball tournament, the company gets, for all intents and purposes, free advertising throughout the game. Every time someone looks at the court, they see the Nike swoosh on the players. That type of marketing and the product credibility that comes from using elite athletes is invaluable. Why not make them pay the athlete's who are gaining this kind of exposure for them? I propose changing the NCAA rules to allow athletes to endorse sport specific products for a limited amount of money, provided that they meet certain academic requirements.

Allowing athletes to endorse sport specific products would solve many of the issues plaguing Division I college athletics. First, it would give athletes an opportunity to earn some type of monetary compensation for their athletic abilities. As Mike Radja noted when asked if he felt that there were some athletes who felt that their scholarship was not enough compensation for their athletic efforts, he said that "I think there are athletes that think that way." Next, by saving the money coming from an outside source, the effect on student athlete relationships would be minimal, as there would be no extra benefits coming from the schools. All of the money would come from the companies who are already cashing in on the ability of the athletes that use their products. Radja noted as well that representatives from these companies actively seek out players to wear their gear, so it would not be a stretch to ask the companies to pay the athletes for their efforts.

By allowing the athletes to endorse the product, they would in turn be able to do some promotional work for the company involved, such as appear in a limited amount of commercials or promotions. This would increase the amount of exposure for the company, which they would undoubtedly be excited about. In addition, this system would allow the NCAA to clamp down on payments from boosters to athletes, which has been a major focus of the organization. By providing a means for athletes to get paid, the NCAA would be justified in creating harsher punishments for athletes who still seek increased outside compensation, which would most likely lead to a drop in the amount of illegal payments accepted by athletes. By placing academic and conduct restrictions on those who would be eligible for endorsements it would encourage athletes who want to seek compensation to act as a model both in and out of the classroom. Finally, by making the payment come from an outside source, the possibility for compensation is opened to athletes at all schools, not only ones with revenue producing sports. There are enough product manufacturers that track athletes, or soccer players, or any athlete in a less popular sport would have an opportunity to be compensated. Overall, this system creates the best balance between maintaining the ideals of the amateur, student athlete and accepting the modern environment of college sports.

Clearly, the world of Division I college sports is one that plays a prominent role in our society. Athletes serve as role models, examples, and friends. The modern college athlete has to balance hours of practice with the course load of a regular student, all the while watching other people make money off of their hard work. Given the amount of money that is both invested in and made off of college sports, it seems clear that the athletes who are creating this highly sought after product should benefit from their work. When thinking of a solution to this problem, it is important to keep in mind the things that make college sports special, such as the appeal of amateurism, the relationship between students and athletes, and the fact that athletes are playing for the love of the game and not for a salary. Keeping these considerations in mind, the ideal situation to this problem would be to allow athletes to endorse sport specific products for a limited fee, provided that they meet certain academic and conduct standards deemed necessary by the NCAA. Doing this will allow the athletes to benefit from their hard work while still keeping the ideals of college sports intact, in a way that is fair to all parties involved. This solution will create an athletic environment with the highest quality of amateur sport possible, which is truly the goal of every fan of college athletics.

Works Cited

Glasser, Jeff. *US News*. 18 Mar. 2002. 4 Mar. 2005 <http://www.us-news.com/usnews/edu/college/sports/articles/18bucks.htm>.

Goff, Brian. "Effects of University Athletics on the University: A Review and Extension of Empirical Assessment." *Journal of Sport Management* 14 (2000): 85-105.

2004-05 NCAA Division I Manual. 2004.

"QB Must Sit Another Game, Make Restitution." 20 Mar. 2005. Associated Press. 2 Apr. 2005 <http://espn.com>.

Radja, Mike. Online interview. 30 Mar. 2005.

"Representative NFL Stadium Public/Private Partnership." Horrow Sports Ventures.

Rovell, Darren. "Multiple Small Deals Beat One Big One." 6 Mar. 2005. 2 Apr. 2005 <http://espn.com>.

Suggs, Welch. "Big Money in College Sports Flows to the Few." *Chronicle of Higher Education* 51 (2004): A46-A49.

Stein, Andrew. *CNN Money*. 8 Mar. 2002. 19 Mar. 2005 <http://money.cnn.com/2002/03/08/companies/hoops_nike/>.

Whiteside, Kelly. "College Athletes Want Cut of Action." *USA Today* 1 Sept. 2004. EBSCO. 29 Mar. 2005

14

Paper or Plastic?

Jessi Wood

In today's society, it is somewhat comical how much importance is given to certain objects. A perfect example is plastic. Now, most people do not think twice about throwing away plastic silverware or chewing on a plastic pen cap, however, cut the plastic into a small rectangle, stamp some numbers into it, design the front of it with a famous painting or nature scene, and place a magnetic stripe on the back and you have one of the most important objects in some people's lives: a credit card. Although a credit card seems like the ultimate method of payment, it is not. Credit cards do not work the way children think they do; it does not let you buy things for free when you have no cash to pay with. It does, however, trick you into thinking you can buy things for free. Unfortunately, credit cards, along with just about every other luxury item in life today, comes with consequences. Credit cards can have negative and detrimental effects, especially to young adults, by feeding shopping addictions, enabling debt, and contributing to the establishment of poor credit.

Credit cards can not be officially deemed as the factor that causes shopping addictions, however, they certainly provide the adequate equipment to feed such addictions. Shopping can definitely be labeled as one of America's favorite pastimes, which is not thought of as negative as long as it is done in moderation. Once the shopping sprees become more frequent and more expensive, however, it often turns into a shopping addiction. Shopping addictions are real and serious problems, just as addiction to drugs and alcohol are. These shopping addictions would not be able to survive once the shoppers funds were depleted, but with credit cards, there is the ability to shop and make purchases to fulfill the addict's cravings, even without having any cash in their pockets or money in their bank accounts. This addiction has a very high rate in the world of recent college graduates. Lorrin Koran, a Stanford psychiatrist said most of the shopaholics he sees "develop their addictions in their early twenties, not long after they got their first real jobs" and first credit cards" (Futrelle).

This is a very sensible time for a shopping addiction to set in. Even if the shopper had a credit card as a college student, the addiction most likely did not really set in until after receiving a degree. This is due to the fact that many college students realize they do not have a decent income coming in regularly enough to afford these sprees, however, the college graduates, many with their first full-time jobs, are now receiving paychecks larger than they've ever received before and begin indulging in the wonders of shopping. This is where a credit card can really start to destroy a person. The shopper, knowing his or her steady income will be able to pay off the purchase made, will "charge it." The recent college graduate, with the steady paycheck, feels they have the ability to purchase anything they want, because for many this is the first time they have ever been financially secure. The first few purchases soon lead to frequent shopping sprees, which soon turn into insatiable cravings to make purchases and spend more money. By having these credit cards to use, the shoppers are able to hide the amounts of money they are actually using to feed this addiction, at least for a little while. However, once the addiction sets in, the compulsive shopper will not be able to stop, and soon credit cards will begin maxing out, and more credit cards will be applied for and soon, that once very generous, financially pleasing, steady income will not even be close to being large enough to feed the addiction, never mind paying off credit card balances. This addiction, which was fed by the ability to "charge it" soon leads to detrimental effects on the shoppers physical and emotional state of well-being. According to Rick Zehr, the vice president of addiction and behavioral services at the Illinois Institute for Addiction Recovery:

> [Relationship] impairment can occur because the person spends time away from home to shop, covers up debt with deception, and emotionally and physically starts to isolate themselves from others as they become preoccupied with their behavior. (Hatfield)

Zehr is explaining how the actions of an addicted shopper really do result in detrimental effects on the shopper's life. As he stated, the addicted shopper begins spending more and more time shopping and feeding their addiction, rather than spending time with others. This addiction, however, simply started out as a college graduate having the ability to purchase an item and thinking they have the ability, and most importantly, the control to put it on a credit card. On the contrary though, once the negative effects of charging purchases to credit cards come into play, it is the credit card companies and the shopping addictions who begin taking control over the shopper.

Credit card users, both compulsive and healthy, are at very high risk to experience debt at a young age. It almost seems that upon being accepted into college, you also make a transition into the world of credit cards. Right around the time you receive your acceptance letters, you also begin to receive applications for credit cards. According to information from NewsTarget.com, eighty percent of students have at least one credit card, and many begin getting into debt during their freshman year. ("Senate Approves"). Much of this is due to the fact that many college students are already in debt. After paying college tuition, room and board, and having to take out college loans, there is generally very little money left to pay for other day-to-day expenses. This is where the credit card can really come into play. The transition from working a part-time job after school in high school, to entering college where most money that had been saved up gets depleted is a traumatic experience. By having a credit card, the student low on cash has a method of payment that requires no immediate cash, and therefore feels much more in control. However, credit cards trick students into believing they can charge things now on their cards, and then just pay it off when they have the cash. This is not really true though. Annual percentage rates for purchases and late fees are placed on credit cards specifically for this purpose. According to student credit card research, only twenty-five percent of students with credit cards paid off their balance each month. That means, seventy-five percent of student credit card holders carried some amount of debt. ("Student Credit Card"). The twenty-five percent that pay off the balance every month are using a credit card to its full advantage and benefiting greatly from its services, however, twenty-five percent represents a minority. The majority of students are the seventy-five percent that have accumulated debt. Therefore, it is the majority of students who are experiencing the negative and detrimental effects of credit cards. Credit cards, however, do a great job enticing students to first of all apply for, and then use the credit cards by offering rewards and benefits with purchases. For example, Citi, a common credit card company, had people go around door-to-door asking students to apply for the card. Upon applying, the student was given a free T-shirt which gives filling out the application that much more appeal. Also, on the front page of the application in bold lettering, it reads, "Use your card. Earn the rewards." The front page goes on to state that by using a Citi card to buy airline tickets the shopper will save fifteen percent off the total and by using it at supermarkets, drugstores, and gas stations the shopper will receive a five percent cash back rate. Now, to a college student low on finances, this may seem like a great offer, however, even though the card is allotting discounts and cash back, the purchase is still being made, and there will still be a balance that must be paid and fees attached to this balance. This is where the student shopper begins to forget the responsibilities that come along with making the purchase and only focuses on the perks. Once this starts happening, the student begins spending money he really does not have, and soon finds himself in debt.

Going almost hand-in-hand with debt is the idea that credit cards also have the ability to create bad credit attached to a person's name. As Jane Bryant Quinn declares in her article titled "Capital Ideas"

> Lenders report all payments to credit bureaus so [you] start building a personal credit history. A good one will help when [you] get out of school. But, if [you] miss payments or pay late, [you] can wreck [yourself] for years. (E26)

In saying this, Quinn is describing how serious credit really is. There is no mother or father in these situations to give second chances or teacher to give extensions, there are only lenders and credit bureaus that have each credit card owner as a name and number on a list. What list the owner is put on is solely dependent upon the actions and history of the card owner. It is a difficult task to maintain a spot on the "good credit list," however, it is doubly as difficult to get off of the "bad credit list." This is a very common problem with college students and recent graduates who are also credit card owners. One example of this scenario is Juanda Smith, a twenty-eight year old woman who currently earns sixty thousand dollars a year. However, Smith is haunted by the bad credit she accumulated during her years as a computer science student at Spelman College. The bad credit haunts her so badly she had difficulties after graduating renting an apartment and getting utilities hooked up. Smith admits, "I didn't understand the big picture of credit. I'd say 'Oh, I forgot to pay this week.' Then a week turns into a month, and a month turns into two months" (Fetterman). Smith is not alone in this situation, this is the case for many young credit card owners. Many do not realize how quickly bad credit can occur, simply by skipping or postponing payments, or even if they do realize the consequences of having a "black mark" on their credit, they do not understand how detrimental the effects will be on their life. Like in Smith's case, students who graduate and begin looking for apartments and houses and have accumulated bad credit history will soon face many hardships, and will quickly realize how serious the issue of credit truly is. The destruction of credit and its negative effects directly relate back to credit cards. It's these credit cards that are allowing students to purchase objects without physically paying money, and then postpone or neglect payments on the balance. In doing this, the negative and detrimental effects of bad credit are overpowering the once beneficial credit card usage.

After analyzing cases of addictive shopping, debt, and bad credit history, and being able to trace all three back to credit card usage only forces people to associate credit cards with negative and detrimental effects. For the majority of credit card users, it creates a vicious cycle they get trapped into. As a broke college student, they apply for a credit card and claim the rewards that really enticed them in, then they use the credit card to make purchases simply because discounts or special offers are associated with usage, however, when the bill comes in the mail and shows the balance that has accumulated the student or former student is unable to pay the balance, or decides to postpone the payment, and continues making further purchases on the card, and can even lead to addictive and compulsive shopping. This not only racks up the balance, but also puts the student or former student into debt, which directly attaches the label of having bad credit. Once the student or former student finds themselves in this scenario, it is near impossible to get out, and even with assistance and guidance on getting out of this horrible nightmare, it takes a great deal of time in order to dissociate the bad history and create new, better credit.

Works Cited

"Citi." Citibank, 2005.

Fetterman, Mindy. "Good Education, Good Job, Bad Credit." *USA Today* 25 Apr. 2005

Futrelle, David . "Do You Shop Too Much?" 31 Oct. 2003. *CNN*. 1 May 2005 <http://money.cnn.com/2003/10/31/pf/shopaholics/>.

Hatfield, Heather. "Shopping Spree, or Addiction?" 2005. *WebMD Health*. 1 May 2005 <http://webcenter.health.webmd.netscape.com/content/article/97/104241.htm>.

Quinn, Jane B. "Capital Ideas." *Newsweek* 21 Mar. 2005: E26.

"Senate Approves Bill Restricting Credit Card Marketing to College Students." 3 May 2005. *News Target*. <http://www.newstarget.com/006536.html>.

"Student Credit Card Research Update." *National On-Campus Report* 15 Oct. 2004: 5.

15

SUV's Confrontational Relationship with Nature and Humans

Christopher Parker

The new Hummer H2 weighs in at a hefty four and a half tons (gross vehicle weight), has a thirty-two gallon gas tank capacity, averages 10.7 miles per gallon (MPG), and has an estimated full tank mileage of less than 350 miles (Heilig). The new Hummer H2 and other sport utility vehicles (SUVs) just like it are responsible for accelerating already existing environmental problems. In 1985, SUVs accounted for only two percent of new vehicles sales. SUVs now account for one in four new vehicles sold, and sales continue to climb (Naughton). Driving an SUV has a much greater impact on the environment and our health than driving other passenger cars. Current federal regulations allow SUVs to have far worse fuel economy than other vehicles. The federal corporate average fuel economy (CAFE) standards set the fuel economy goals for new passenger cars at 27.5 mpg. Light trucks only have to achieve 20.7 mpg ("Environmental Double Standards"). Most SUVs are so large that they don't fit into either of these categories and are not subjected to any kind of fuel economy standards (Goewey 120). The benefits of owning an SUV are not worth the impact they make on the environment and our health because the amount of gasoline they use increases the threat of global warming, increases smog forming emissions, and contributes to the demise of the world's already limited oil resources.

It seems like almost overnight SUVs have invaded our roadways. These vehicles are capable of going on safaris deep into the woods, yet why are these seemingly benign vehicles beginning to populate even our most urban of roadways? In an essay by David Grasso titled "SUVs: Devils in Disguise," he says that "SUVs are roomy, safe for occupants, and convenient, I thought SUVs were God's gift to the American roadway" (Grasso). These three reasons seem to be the only benefits associated with owning an SUV in today's ever growing urban world. It is indisputable that SUVs are extremely roomy with three rows of seating capable of carrying seven to nine passengers. They even have the capacity to fold down all of the rear seats for cargo room that on average can exceed 100 cubic feet ("SUVs").

It is also true that when it comes to protection, people who own SUVs are traveling in one of the safest vehicles on the road as compared to those traveling in compacts cars. This is mostly a result of their gigantic size and weight. The extra weight of SUVs rearranges where the deaths occur in crashes, transferring deaths from SUVs to the cars. In accordance with this, a study by the National Highway Safety Traffic Administration says that in an accident involving a car and an SUV, the occupants of the car are 3.4 times more likely to be killed than if they had been hit by another car. One reason is a simple law of physics. When two vehicles collide, the one with more mass wins (Koloff). It is clear that occupants in SUVs are much safer compared to those traveling in compact cars.

Along with being very roomy and safe, SUVs are very convenient. Almost every SUV comes with two-wheel drive, four-wheel drive, and all-wheel drive. They also offer several convenient standard options, including climate control, heated seats, power door locks, power windows, power seats, telescoping steering wheel, CD players with CD changers that can hold in excess of 10 CDs, and also include such things as colored navigation displays with talking directions. These are all very convenient items available in SUVs today and the list continues to grow with time. The benefits of SUVs being roomy, safe for the occupants, and convenient all seem very minute, however, when we take into account the amount of gasoline they use and the impact that this has on our environment and our health everyday.

The amount of gasoline used by an SUV is important for several reasons. One of the most important is the threat of global warming. Every gallon of gasoline a vehicle burns puts 20 pounds of carbon dioxide (CO_2) into the atmosphere. Today a car that gets approximately 27.5 mpg, like a new Volkswagen Beetle, will emit 54 tons of carbon dioxide from the burning of gasoline over its lifetime. An SUV that averages 14 mpg, like the Hummer H2, will emit over 100 tons of carbon dioxide over its lifetime. This means that a full-size SUV can emit up to twice a much carbon dioxide per mile as the average car ("Environmental Double"). According to the Environmental Protection Agency (EPA), the high levels of carbon dioxide released by these SUVs are causing an increase in concentrations of greenhouse gases (water vapor, carbon dioxide, and other gases) causing an acceleration in the rate of climate change. Scientists expect that the average global surface temperature could rise 1 degree to 4.5 degrees Fahrenheit in the next fifty years, and 2.2 to 10 degrees in the next century (EPA). This will result in much more unfavorable climates to live in, especially countries close to the equator with already very hot climates. This increased temperature could potentially cause deaths to infants and the elderly who are extremely susceptible to the body stresses caused by heat. Evaporation will also increase as the temperature climbs, which will increase average global precipitation. Soil moisture is likely to decline in many regions due to this evaporation (EPA). This will result in decreased farming productivity due to lack of areas with enough moisture to actually grow any type of crop. Increased evaporation will also most likely cause intense rainstorms to become more frequent (EPA). These intense rainstorms have a possibility of causing an increase in devastating floods causing billions of dollars in damage and the deaths of vegetation, animals, and most important, humans. The sea level is likely to rise two feet along most of the U.S. coast line (EPA). It is evident that global warming is a dangerous threat to the entire world and should not be ignored. However, automakers continue to build fuel-inefficient SUVs that are accelerating the world problem of global warming. The benefits associated with these SUVs do not compare to the devastation that the world will face if something isn't done about the fuel inefficiencies of these vehicles.

SUVs also have a significant environmental impact beyond global warming. SUVs emit large quantities of smog forming emissions. Sport utility vehicles can put out thirty percent more carbon monoxide and hydrocarbons and seventy-five percent more nitrogen oxides than passenger cars ("Environmental Double"). These combustion pollutants contribute to eye and throat irritation, coughing, nausea, dizziness, fatigue, confusion, and headaches. Hydrocarbons and nitrogen oxides are precursors to ground level ozone, which causes asthma and lung damage (Wagner 88-103). All passenger vehicles pollute, but SUVs produce a much larger amount of pollution than the average car. In terms of air pollution, one SUV equals two or three cars on the road. The SUVs producing these smog-forming emissions are obviously more hazardous to our health than compared to compact cars. The benefits of SUVs don't compare with the health hazards that they cause.

Along with global warming and emitting enormous amounts of smog forming emissions, SUVs are responsible in part for the dwindling amount of the world's oil reserves due to their low fuel economy. The Environmental Protection Agency says that America accounts for five percent of the world's population, but we consume twenty-five percent of the world's oil, or 20 million barrels of oil a day (EPA). If current rates of consumption were to continue, the world's remaining resources of conventional oil would be used up in forty years ("Annual Energy"). This evidence proves that there will be no gasoline for future generations if our SUVs continue to consume it at twelve miles per gallon. It's also true that for the most part oil is a non-renewable source meaning that once it is gone, it is gone practically forever. A staggering ninety-eight tons of pre-historic, buried plant material—or 196,000 pounds—along with an extensive amount of time is required to produce each gallon of gasoline we burn in our cars, SUVs, trucks, and other vehicles, according to a study conducted at the University of Utah ("Bad Mileage"). It is terrible to think that SUVs are responsible for the demise of the world's oil, yet according to David Goewey in an essay entitled "Careful, You May Run Out of Planet," the SUV is the fastest-growing segment of the automobile market (113). This is scary knowing that the world will soon run out of oil if it does not do something about the miles per gallon that current SUVs get. We risk this all at the expense of having a vehicle that is roomy, safer for the occupants, and more convenient. Considering the amount of cars on the road, an increase in efficiency of SUVs of even a few miles per gallon of gasoline can save over a million barrels of oil a day ("Annual Energy"). By reducing the amount of oil we use currently, we are conserving the rapidly dwindling natural resource for future generations caused largely in part by SUVs.

It is clear to see that owning a SUV is certainly not worth killing our planet along with ourselves at the same time. SUVs, due to their poor fuel economy, are rapidly diminishing the world's oil reserves, increasing the threat of global warming, and increasing smog forming emissions while owners of these vehicles are only benefiting from the mere fact that they are roomy, safe, and convenient. All of these are hazardous to the human race and the earth as we know it. If something isn't done about the SUV craze in America and around the world, everyone is going to suffer. Is ruining our health and destroying the earth we live on worth owning these SUVs?

Works Cited

"Annual Energy Review 2000." *Energy Information Administration*. 2000. 2 May 2005. <http://www.eia.doe.gov>.

"Bad Mileage: 98 Tons of Plants per Gallon." *University of Utah News and Public Relations*. 27 October, 2003. 2 May 2005. <http://www.utah.edu/unews/releases/03/oct/gas.html>.

"Environmental Double Standards for Sport Utility Vehicles." 2002. 2 May 2005. <http://www.suv.or/environ.html>.

EPA, Global Warming. *Environmental Protection Agency.* 7 January, 2000. 2 May 2005. <http://Yosemite.epa.gov/oar/globalwarming.nsf/content/Climate.html>.

Goewey, David. "'Careful, You May Run Out of Planet': SUVs and the Exploitation of the American Myth." *Signs of Life in the USA: Readings on Popular Culture for Writers,* 4th ed. Ed. Sonia Maasik and Jack Solomon. New York: Bedford/St. Martin's, 2003. 112-126.

Grasso, David. "SUVs: Devils in Disguise." 14 February 2003. *The Sandspur.* 3 May 2005. <http://wwww.thesandspur.org/news/2003/02/14/Opinions/Suvs-Devils.In.Disguise-373089.html>.

Heilig, John. "2003 Hummer H2 Road Test." *Family Car.* 2002. 2 May 2005. <http://www.familycar.com/RoadTests/Hummer H2/>.

Koloff, Abbott. "Debate rages on benefit of owning SUVs." *Daily Record News.* 8 February 2004. 1 May 2005. <http://www.dailyrecord.com/news/articles/news3-aksuvs.htm>.

Naughton, Keith. "The Unstoppable SUV." *Newsweek.* July 2, 2001.

"SUVs, What You Should Know Before You Buy." *Edmunds.* 2005. 3 May 2005. <http://www.edmunds.com/buyguide/suv.html>.

Wagner, Travis. *In Our Backyard: A guide to understanding pollution and its effects.* New York: Reinhold, 1994.

16

The Future of the Corporate World

Lisa McElheny

As we stare down the tunnel of our future we are drawing closer to the "real world" with every breathe we take. Higher education enrollment numbers have increased rapidly and, in the increasingly competitive business world, having a bachelor's degree hardly gets you in the door. The demands for MBAs, masters, PhDs, and diverse educational experience are skyrocketing. How will you stand out? Is a degree enough? What makes you unique? For most of us the point of college is to advance our education and experience in a specific field, suggesting a move away from diversification. However, diversification is beneficial to any job seeking graduate; any quality that places you one step ahead of your competition can make all the difference. The answer for worrisome college students across the country is bilingual abilities. With immigrant numbers on the rise and a business world which is becoming more multicultural everyday, the need for bilingual employees is higher than ever (Shin and Bruno 185). Being multilingual is an asset in the workplace, and one that is being met with increasing compensation.

Though disputed by many favoring the English only mentality, bilingual career advancement is evident in multiple cases throughout my research. Though undisputedly related, I am not engaging in the controversial debate of the English language in the United States, but suggesting the advantages bilingualism has in our corporate world. This progression can be established not only in international jobs, but those operating within our borders. Through theories, examples, and extrinsic proof I plan to establish bilingual applicants as superior within the work force.

Though the basis of my argument states that being bilingual advances careers in our modern business world, there is the basic assumption of English proficiency. Even without English as our established national language it is shared as the common ground for communication within our society. The term bilingual within the United States currently identifies fluency in English with an additional language understanding. For Veronica Sanchez, local news reporter in Nevada, her Spanish-speaking abilities have allowed her to cover Hispanic stories, yet the majority of her work assignments still require proficiency in English (Whitney 12). In order for an employee or applicant to benefit from multilingual assets they must also have the necessary English communication skills to work in our English dominated population.

In chart after chart of the 2000 Census one concept was eminent: minorities are on the rise (Shin and Bruno 185). This increase in the number of immigrants entering our society directly connects to another Census chart depicting the number of foreign tongues spoken in the United States (Shin and Bruno 185). Though many argue over theoretical subtext of this situation and the implications the entry of these minorities may have, the business world sees it in a much simpler mindset. The increase in minorities and foreign languages can be simply stated as profit, and businesses across the country are adapting to meet this growing market. From 1990 to 2000 the number of non-English speaking people grew by over 15 million (Shin and Bruno 185). As minorities in our country rapidly increase and the numbers for non-English speaking citizens grow, language and communication barriers are becoming increasingly complicated. Though there is a continual need for bilingual employees in international business, our recent minority trends depicted in the 2000 Census have created a need for multilingual services and workers within our American borders.

As diverse language populations continue to increase so does the demand for bilingual business practices and employees. In recent years the need for bilingual business operations has become increasingly imminent. ATMs now offer a variety of language instructions, telephone service operations begin with a language option, and the number of Spanish-speaking TV channels are on the rise (Whitney 12). The advantage in offering these services is the company's ability to reach the largest number of potential consumers. The hidden factor behind the operations of any business is its employees, and the demand for multilingual production services is directly connected to the increased demand for a bilingual staff. The 2000 Census claimed seventeen percent of Nevada is Hispanic; this development has forced local TV stations to face their changing market (Shin and Bruno 186). With an obligation to communicate to their region news director for KRNV, an NBC affiliate, Jon Killoran has felt pressure to modify their existing operations (Whitney 12-13). He now identifies bilingual abilities as a prominent factor in the hiring of new applicants, and that this skill has had mounting importance over the past few years (Whitney 12-13). Killoran and the KRNV station are perfect examples that the increase of non-English speaking citizens has directly heightened the need for bilingual services and regional employee's to administer them.

In my research one of the most promising pieces of evidence was through a simple job search on a well-known internet site known as Monster.com. Anyone can easily access this site and simply type in a region, interest, or skill which then generates a list of all job opportunities relevant to your information. Once at Monster.com, I simply typed "bilingual" as a keyword and found twenty pages of job opportunities and companies looking for applicants with this skill. Jane Rifkin, editor of *Hispanic Times Magazine*, recently wrote that health care, finance, government, and manufacturing firms were the fields with the greatest demand for bilingual employees (10). I found this statement was overwhelmingly evident in my job search. The site displays requests for multicultural and multilingual applicants from a wide range of high-profile corporations such as Bank of America, Verizon Wireless, and Time Warner Cable. With daily updates of over 1,000 bilingual jobs, Monster.com offers extrinsic proof of the overwhelming demand for multicultural and bilingual applicants.

Business has also been reshaped by the significant growth of the international market. Companies across the country are realizing that international markets are profitable, and the cultural and physical boundaries that once enclosed societies are quickly retreating. This rapid loss of international limitations has intensified the need for cultural diversity and understanding in the workplace. For a company to market an "American" product overseas, it first must identify with that culture by recognizing what their values and needs are. McDonalds, for example, has unique menus for each region it serves and adapts its products and techniques based on the societies they are advertising to. For companies in this lucrative international business, employees that can carry out international operations can determine a corporation's success.

Stephen Steinburg, author of "The Cultural Fallacy in Studies of Ethnic Mobility," identifies that culture is what separates us as people (61). Though language significantly affects societal differences, a further identifier in what diversifies the universal population is culture. Applying this concept to our modern business world suggests that successful international business is significantly dependent on cultural adaptations. For many global companies the tools behind global profits are employees who are culturally diverse and able to identify with their customer base. In recent years the well known Microsoft Encarta has reshaped its concept in order to appeal to diverse cultures (Kohlmeier 2). In order to effectively target each regions beliefs and values they not only look for bilingual employees but more importantly those who have multicultural backgrounds. Microsoft found that in order to sell to a new market, they first had to identify the needs and wants within that market (Kohlmeier 10). They were able to adapt their product by hiring employees with cultural understanding of their customer base, and in doing so they could more efficiently satisfy customers, and ultimately increase sales. Though being bilingual improves job opportunities, being culturally diverse can have similar affects. With hundreds of big businesses such as McDonalds and Microsoft becoming multidimensional, the need for diverse operations and the opportunities for multicultural employees are skyrocketing.

In both foreign and domestic markets career options for bilingual applicants are rapidly expanding and this new demand is being met with increasing compensation. Having employees who are able to speak multiple languages is beneficial to the company and these employees are looking for a wage increase to effectively meet their contributions. Peter Fritsch, staff reporter for *The Wall Street Journal*, analyzed the request from Southwest Bell employees who feel their multilingual knowledge should be met with higher wages (A1). Fritsch looks at bilingual employees as any other product in the corporate world, "it's simply supply and demand," what is in higher demand is economically valuable and often more expensive (A1). In relation to the bilingual market the demand for workers with this ability is greater than the supply and with their growing value employees are expecting the compensation they feel they deserve. Fritsch's theory is being put to actual use in hundreds of company's across the country feeling the pressure from foreign and domestic minority markets.

In October 2001 the city of Lubbock was forced to respond to the 28.5 percent of its population who are Spanish speaking ("Lubbock" 3). A policy was passed which required all companies to include a monthly forty-dollar increase in wages for all employees who are bilingual ("Lubbock" 3). Lubbock is not alone in this language reward; other Texas cities such as Waco, Fort Worth, Grand Prairie and Carrollton are also increasing salaries for bilingual employees ("Lubbock" 3). "As the nation's demographics change, cities across America will find it advantageous to monetarily reward employees for their [multilingual] abilities," claims Victor Hernandez the president of Hispanic Elected Local Officials ("Lubbock" 3). Though Lubbock currently only offers this monthly stipend for Spanish-speaking individuals who pass an oral assessment they have already recognized that if the need for other languages increases they are willing to offer the current pay increase to others with similar multilingual capabilities.

Texas' demand for Spanish to be incorporated into business operations is easily connected to its physical boundaries; however bilingual compensation is not limited to Hispanic dominated populations. Jane Rifkin, *Hispanic Times Magazine* editor, adds that the Los Angeles city school district, as well as many other districts, presents a $5,000 salary increase for all bilingual employees (10). In addition, Rifkin points out that all multilingual employees at Kaiser Permanente receive higher salaries by about five percent than unilingual workers (10). With international and minority markets on the rise the compensation for these abilities could be the future of our corporate world.

The effects of this business transition are already being felt by the educational world. In most high school districts a language is required for a number of years culminating with an equivalency exam. Although that is the end of bilingual education for most, the emphasis on extended multilingual comprehension is rapidly advancing. Currently UNH offers a duel major program in international affairs; this unique program promotes students to receive a degree in their field of choice with an additional degree in international study. In order to complete this degree the university requires and eight-week study in another country and complete comprehension of a foreign language. Complete understanding of a foreign language will only help a graduate in their career search; however students can reap some of the benefits by even being diverse educationally and culturally. As the business world continues to be revamped, educational opportunities across the country are close behind. The need for diverse education as well as multicultural and multilingual abilities are greater than ever.

Through my extensive research it is evident that diversity and multicultural understanding are the future of the corporate world. With the significant need for bilingual employees both for our minority markets in the United States, as well as international markets the demand for workers with these capabilities is undisputable. In addition to the request for multilingual applicants, the city of Lubbock displayed the considerable rewards offered for these skills. As Jane Rifkin stated, "it's not what you do as much as who you are" (10). Mastering English plus one and becoming cultural adaptable makes any applicant a more marketable employee and an asset to any business in today's increasingly international commercial world.

Works Cited

Fritsch, Peter. "Bilingual Employees Are Seeking More Pay, and May Now get it." *Wall Street Journal* 288: 96 (1996): A1.

Kohlmeier, Bernhard. "Microsoft Encarta Goes Multilingual." *Translating Into Success*. Ed. Roberts Sprung. Philadelphia: John Benjamins Publishing Company, 2000. 1-11.

Litvan, Laura. "Casting a Wider Employment Net" *Nation's Business* 82: 12 (1994): 49-54.

"Lubbock Gives Bonus to Bilingual Employees." *Nation's Cities Weekly* 25: 18 (2002): 3.

Monster Networking. 2004. Monster Job Search. 18 April 2005 <http://jobsearch.monster.com/jobsearch>.

Rifkin, Jane. "Letter from the editor: The competitive edge." *Hispanic Times Magazine* 17: 1 (1996): 10.

Shin, Hyon B. and Rosalind Bruno. "Census 2000: Language Use and English-Speaking Ability in the United States." *What's Language Got to do With It?* New York: W.W. Norton & Company, 2005. 181-196.

Steinburg, Stephen. "The Cultural Fallacy in Studies of Racial and Ethnic Mobility." *Immigrants, Schooling and Social Mobility*. Ed. Hans Vermeulen. London: Macmillan Press Ltd., 2000. 61-71.

Whitney, Daisy. "Bilingual Reporters Have the Inside Track" *Electronic Media* 21: 33 (2002): 12-13.

17

Single-Parent Homes: Quality, Not Quantity

Jessica DiStefano

In recent years, many families have been diverging from the traditional family structure and adopting different ones such as single-parent homes, single-parent co-habiting homes, divorced and remarried homes, and multigenerational families. Many people believe that when children are raised in single-parent homes they are less apt to be successful academically. The thinking is that single-parents have a lower income, so they cannot provide certain resources the child needs for school. Also, the parent has less time to spend with her children and less time to engage in school-associated events. Our culture is biased against single-parent homes and place a certain stigma around them. This stigma attached to single-parent homes then places a certain stereotype around the children from these homes Many people in our society think that there is something wrong with single-parent homes and the children that come from these homes. I have felt that stigma growing up in a single-parent home. However, contrary to what these critics think, I have been very successful academically, graduating from high school in the top ten of my class and continuing on to attend the honors program at the University of New Hampshire. While the critics' reasoning has some validity, research indicates that the number of parents in the home does not determine whether or not the child will be successful. Rather, it is the relationship the parent has with the child as well as individual family structure and mother's education level that determine the child's academic success.

The number of children living in single-parent homes is increasing and is projected to continue to increase in the upcoming years. The 2002 Current Population Survey reveals that sixty-nine percent of children under eighteen lived with two parents, twenty-three percent of children under eighteen lived with their mother only, and five percent of children under eighteen lived with their father only (Fields 3). Single-parent homes are the result of divorce, death, or unwed families with the number of single unwed families contributing the most to the single-parent population

(Jeynes 74). It is estimated that about fifty to sixty percent of all children born in the 1990s will spend some time living in a single-parent home before they reach the age of eighteen (Deleire and Kalil 394). By 1993, the percentage of children under eighteen not living with both biological parents was forty-three percent (Jeynes 74), and according to the 2000 census, single-parent homes account for twenty-eight percent of households with children (Deleire and Kalil 394). Since the number of children being raised in single-parent homes is increasing it is important to look at the effects that these single-parent homes may have on children.

One reason critics believe that children living in single-parent homes tend to do worse academically than those who come from intact homes is the socioeconomic standing of the family. According to Henry Ricciuti, "in 1998 the median family income for single mothers with children under 18 years was $16,326, and 47% of those children fell below the poverty level; comparable figures for two-parent families were $52,553 and 9% respectively" (196). This level of socioeconomic distress leads to decreased resources for school needs. Research has found that "family economic resources account for half the differences in child development outcomes between single-mother families and their two-parent counterparts" (Deleire and Kalil 395). Studies have also found that students from single-parent or stepfamilies are three times more likely to drop out of school than those students who come from two parent homes, even after socioeconomic status and ability have been taken into account (Lee and Zimiles 317). Differences in income also account for thirty to fifty percent of the differences in high school graduation rates between those from intact families and those not (Astone and McLanahan 309). Decreased income, along with the single-parent's lack of time, are two of the main reasons people feel that children from single-parent homes are at an educational disadvantage.

Single parents must work longer hours than those parents in two-parent households, thus decreasing the amount of time left to monitor schoolwork, participate in the child's school events, or spend leisure time with the child. Families containing two parents have the advantage of another income and also another parent to spend time with the children. Due to the lack of resources and parental time, single parents may have lower expectations for their child's scholastic achievement (Ricciuti 196). Therefore, students from single-parent homes will be more likely to drop out of school than those from intact homes. Ricciuti found that "the educational attainment of young adults in their mid-20s was found to be associated negatively with time spent in a one-parent family or significantly reduced for participants who lived continuously with a single parent from age 6 to 15" (197). This indicates that a child's educational success will be negatively affected by living in a single-parent home. Not only is the parent's lack of time detrimental to a child's educational attainment, but it also could be negatively associated with the child's social development.

A common belief in our society is that two parents are necessary for effective child rearing and that children from single-parent homes do not receive consistent child rearing. Researchers believe that the poor academic achievement of children from single-parent homes is more likely the result of "social deviance" than it is of "cognitive deficiency" (Lee and Zimiles 317). Children from single-parent homes are also more likely to engage in risky behavior such as sex and drug use, which could also be a result of poor child rearing. Therefore, growing up in a single-parent home will negatively affect the child both academically and socially.

My experience contradicts these research findings and leads me to disagree with them. Having grown up in a single-parent home, I believe that a child's academic success is not determined solely by the number of parents present in the home. My father passed away when I was seven and my sister was twelve, and it has been the two of us, along with my mother, ever since. Both my sister and I were involved in rigorous honors classes in high school, graduated and went on to attend four-year colleges. I was secretary of our high school's National Honor Society, graduated seventh in my class of 261 students, was accepted to the honors programs at the University of New Hampshire and the University of Rhode Island, and was offered a Balfour Scholarship to Wheaton College. My mother and two uncles also grew up in a single-parent home after their father passed away when they were young. Their mother had only an eighth grade education and worked in a jewelry factory, but she valued education and had high expectations for her children. She believed that education was the key for her children to have more economic stability than she had. Although my mother and her two brothers were economically disadvantaged these factors did not negatively affect them. My mother went on to receive the highest grade point average of her entire eighth-grade class. She later graduated from high school, college, and graduate school. She received a master's degree in mathematics and is currently a high school mathematics teacher. One of my uncles graduated from high school, attended college, and went on to become a Command Sergeant Major in the National Guard. He currently has a management position at a manufacturing company in our state. My other uncle graduated from high school and went on to graduate from college with a degree in pharmacy. He continued to be a pharmacist for many years until retiring last year. All of these people came from single-parent homes and did not fall victim to the common misconception that they would be academically unsuccessful. This leads me to conclude that the idea that children from single-parent homes are less likely to achieve academic success is a mistaken belief.

While it does hold true that single-parent homes are more likely to be poverty stricken and that there is less time for the parent to spend with the children, these two factors are not the only ones that contribute to academic failure, nor do they preclude the possibility of success. Stepfamilies are, in a sense, equivalent to intact families in that there are two parents supervising and twice the income. However, studies have shown that while children from intact families fare the best, children from stepfamilies do just as poorly as, if not worse than, those children from single-parent homes. Also, when comparing children from single-parent homes and those from stepfamilies researchers found the results for the two groups to be indistinguishable (Lee and Zimiles 317). This supports the idea that two parents are not necessarily better than one. It is also important to note that children in step-parent families have lower educational aspirations and less parental involvement with schoolwork (Astone and McLanahan 315). This evidence refutes the argument that children from single-parent homes do worse academically because the parent does not have enough time to spend with the child. Children from stepfamilies grow up with two parents, as do children from intact families, and still do not receive adequate help with their schoolwork. Research indicates that children from step-parent homes, divorced or widowed remarried homes and blended families all do worse than those children from single-parent homes. This evidence leads me to believe that the number of parents is not the deciding factor of a child's academic success.

One factor that may account for the similar outcomes for children of step-parent and single-parent families is the relationship between the parent and child. When a child lives with only one parent a strong emotional bond develops between the two. However, when the parent remarries this bond is usually lost as the result of either the parent's spending more time with his or her new spouse or the child's resenting the fact that the parent has remarried. A study performed by Valerie E. Lee and Herbert Zimiles found that a child's drop-out behavior is interrelated with the gender of the single parent. Children living with the same gendered parent were less likely to drop out in single-parent families but more likely to drop out in stepfamilies. For example, if a single mother and daughter are living together the probability of the daughter dropping out is very low. However, once a stepfather is brought into the picture, the probability that the daughter will drop out is increased. They also discovered that if the same gendered parent remarries the odds are that the parent's same gendered child is more likely to drop out of school than the parent's opposite gendered child. For example, if a mother remarries, the odds that her daughter will drop out increase while the odds are that her son will drop out decrease (314 & 318). Studies have found that blended families, in which some of the children belong to both parents and some belong to only one, are also more negatively correlated with academic achievement than single-parent families (Ginther and Pollak 684). It seems that even though these families have the same number of parents as traditional families, children are not necessarily better off.

Many people believe that the addition of another caregiver would increase a child's academic success; however this theory is not supported by research. After controlling for variables such as socioeconomic status, race, and gender, studies found that living with a co-habiting couple or a remarried widow(er) had the greatest impact on the academic success of children (Jeynes 73). Children from divorced parents who have remarried perform worse academically than children from divorced parents who have not remarried. The act of remarriage after either divorce or death of a spouse has a negative effect on children's performance on standardized tests (Jeynes 89). Also, a child's risk of being left back a grade increases when the child comes from a widowed remarried family rather than when a child comes from a widowed single-parent family. Likewise, a child from a divorced remarried family also has an increased risk of being left behind a grade when compared to a child from a divorced single-parent family (Jeynes 89). These studies suggest that although another caregiver is present, if that caregiver is non-biological there is a greater negative impact on the academic success of children than there would be for a child from a single-parent home, which does not include the presence of a non-biological caregiver (Jeynes 91-92). Therefore, although they are lacking a parent, children in single-parent homes may be better off than those children in remarried homes.

These differences in children's academic achievement may be influenced more by family dynamics than by the number of adult caregivers present in the home. Two caregivers that are related to the child (i.e., intact families) positively affect the child's academic success, while two caregivers who are not both related to the child negatively affect the child's academic success more than if the child had just one caregiver. This may be due to the adjustment that the child must undergo when the non-biological caregiver enters the family; thus, this adjustment period may lead to the negative outcome. Children from remarried families often face rivalries with their new step-siblings as well as jealous feelings toward their new step-parent. The step-parent may also reduce the close relationship between the child and biological parent (Jeynes 78). Decreased achievement would occur either because the step-parent is less willing to help a child that is not his or her biological child or the child is reluctant to get close to the step-parent and receive the step-parent's affection (Astone and McLanahan 311). The idea that children from single-parent homes do worse academically because of an absent parent and decreased socioeconomic status cannot explain why children from a remarried family do worse than those children from a single-parent family (Jeynes 91). Therefore, these two reasons cannot be the only factors at fault when a child does not perform well academically.

Mother's education is also an important factor when determining the success of children from single-parent homes. Ricciuti notes a study performed by Biblarz and Raftery in which it was reported that "higher levels of maternal education appeared to offset some of the socioeconomic disadvantages associated with living in female-headed households during childhood or adolescence with respect to years of schooling completed" (202). Although single-mother households were poorer than two-parent households, studies have found that these mothers differed very little in levels of ability, education, or expectations for their children. These factors represent important social resources known to positively impact a child's academic success (203). Although they are worse off economically, the presence of maternal or family characteristics such as mother's competence and education as well as positive maternal expectations and attitudes toward children's education, can positively impact children who live in single-parent homes by increasing their development and educational achievement (203). For example, although my grandmother was not well educated, she valued education as a means for obtaining a better life and she conveyed this attitude to her children. After controlling for mother's education and income level, Donna K. Ginther and Robert A. Pollak found that the effects of living in a single-parent home are no longer statistically significant (691). They also discovered that children of widows are equally successful academically as children in traditional two-parent families (696). Children coming from single-parent homes whose mothers are actively engaged in their academic performance are likely to succeed. Although there is a missing parent, if the remaining parent is educated and shows the child the importance of academic success, then the child is not any worse off than those children who come from two-parent families.

Another interesting discovery is that children who grow up in multigenerational families achieve better academically than those children who are in common two-parent families. The 2000 census revealed that 3.7 percent of all homes are multigenerational, meaning that a grandparent is also present in the home. Studies show that children who live in a home with a single parent and at least one grandparent exhibit higher educational outcomes than those children living in a single mother family without a grandparent present (Deleire and Kalil 394). These teens also exhibit educational and developmental outcomes that are the same as, if not greater than, those teens who live in intact families (393). Also, it has been noted that a strong network of close relatives supporting the child positively impacts the academic success of children living with a single mother (394). My experience is consistent with these findings. I come from a close family where my uncles and grandmother take an interest in my academic success. We have dinner together at my grandmother's house every Sunday, allowing us to keep in touch with each other. They attended many of my high-school awards ceremonies and even now that I am away at college they still call me once a week to see how I am and ask how school is going. I believe that this interest they take in my academics has contributed much to my success. Furthermore, children from never-married, single mother, multigenerational families are as likely to graduate from high school and attend college as those children in married families even though the former come from the poorest family structure of all (403). These results support the fact that the socioeconomic status of a single-parent home cannot be blamed for the child's academic failure.

A child's academic success also is influenced more by the way she is brought up than by economic circumstances. Nan Marie Astone and Sarah S. McLanahan state that "success in school among poor children of all family types is related to deliberate efforts on the part of parents to inculcate discipline and good study habits in their children" (311). Interaction and good communication between the parent and the child is a key element for the child's success. Love, affection, and time are also other important factors contributing to child outcomes (Ginther and Pollak 675). The theory that children from single-parent homes are negatively affected because they do not have as much time to spend with their parent is mistaken. Astone and McLanahan found that children in single-parent homes spend significantly more time talking to their parents than children with two parents (318). My experience supports this finding. For the past four years it has been only my mother and me at home, allowing us to spend a lot of time together, resulting in a special closeness between us. I do not think this would have occurred had my father still been alive. Although I would still spend time with my parents, there would be two around instead of one leaving less time for my mother and me to share alone. A study performed by Ginther and Pollak shows that children who live with single parents perform significantly better on reading comprehension tests (690). This may be the result of their spending a significant amount of time communicating with their parent. Therefore, the idea that children from single-parent homes fail because their parents do not spend an adequate amount of time talking with them is wrong. These studies indicate that children from single-parent families do not necessarily perform poorly and sometimes they can perform just as well as children who live with two parents.

Family income and the number of parents in the household are not the only factors that determine a child's academic success. Other factors such as parental involvement and the lack of stress caused by non-biological caregivers can influence how well a child will perform academically. Critics who simply believe that if a child comes from a single-parent home she is less apt to achieve high academic standards are mistaken. Children whose parents have been remarried are less likely to perform well academically than those who come from single-parent homes. It is important to understand that with regard to a child's academic achievement the common phrase "quality not quantity" holds true. Research has found that many factors contribute to a child's academic success and thus the idea that children from single-parent homes are less likely to achieve academically is an old and outdated assumption.

Works Cited/Consulted

Astone, Nan Marie and Sara S. McLanahan. "Family Structure, Parental Practices, and High School Completion." *American Sociological Review* 56.3 (1991): 309-320.

Deleire, Thomas and Ariel Kalil. "Good Things Come in Threes: Single-Parent Multigenerational Family Structure and Adolescent Adjustment." *Demography.* 39.2 (2002): 393-413.

Fields, Jason. "Children's Living Arrangements and Characteristics: March 2002."
United States Census Bureau Current Population Reports. P20-547 (2003): 1-20.

Ginther, Donna K. and Robert A. Pollak. "Family Structure and Children's Educational Outcomes: Blended Families, Stylized Facts, and Descriptive Regressions." *Demography.* 41.4 (2004): 671-696.

Jeynes, William H. "The Effects of Several of the Most Common Family Structures on the Academic Achievement of Eighth Graders." *Marriage and Family Review.* 30.1/2 (2000): 73-97.

Lee, Valerie E. and Herbert Zimiles. "Adolescent Family Structure and Educational Progress." *Developmental Psychology.* 27.2 (1991): 314-320.

Ricciuti, Henry N. "Single Parenthood, Achievement, and Problem Behavior in White, Black, and Hispanic Children." *Journal of Educational Research.* 97.4 (2004): 196-216.

18

Solid Waste Disposal Practices— An Argument for Cost-Effective Recycling

Craig M. Shillaber

Trash. Every human produces and disposes of it daily. In doing so, there are two primary options: first to throw it all into the waste basket and dispose of it accordingly by landfill or incinerator, and second to separate out those items that are recyclable from the regular waste for separate disposal and reuse through recycling. This text will investigate these options in accordance with where these different types of waste go, what the monetary and environmental costs are, and to what extent we should actually incorporate recycling into solid waste disposal practices. It may not be appropriate to recycle all possible materials at this time, thus care should be taken in designing programs that will be successful and viable for the economic and ecological future.

The Origin of the Discussion

Waste disposal and recycling are not new concepts. In reality, they have been a fact of life for as long as men have walked the earth. However, modern recycling is still a young practice. The major push for it came about in the late 1980s, when numerous landfills closed for various reasons ranging from being at full capacity to environmental hazards. The closings brought about the belief that there was a solid waste crisis since many more old landfills were shutting down than new ones were opening. However, this belief was a false presumption since the new landfills were much larger and safer than those that closed, meaning the overall capacity was not actually decreasing, but remaining the same, or in some cases even increasing (Ackerman 19).

Space or availability of disposal facilities was not the only factor contributing to the recycling debate. Several environmental concerns were also raised about disposal practices. These included the impact of emissions from the combustion of waste in incinerators and their affect on the atmosphere, as well as landfill gases and leachate, which will be discussed later.

The conceived solution to these feared problems was modern recycling, which many municipalities quickly began to promote. Public programs were developed across the country, but many suffered economic hardship because often "The costs of collecting, sorting, and baling recyclable materials exceeds the prices that local organizations receive from brokers or remanufacturers" (Weinberg, Pellow and Schnaiberg 44). This means that in some cases, recycling was costing more money to implement than it was earning in the resale of the recovered materials, resulting in an economic drain on municipalities. Naturally, this led to a heated and ongoing debate about whether recycling is even worthwhile. The arguments of both sides are important to understand, and careful evaluation is needed so that the proper decision in caring for and looking to the future may be made.

Landfills, Incineration and the Environment— An Evaluation for Recycling

Landfills are areas of land specifically designated and managed for the disposal of waste. Within their bounds, garbage is literally piled up, compacted and buried. Hence the reason they are so often referred to as "dumps." According to the Environmental Protection Agency's (EPA) web site of Solid Waste Basic Facts, landfilling accounts for fifty-six percent of all solid waste disposal in the United States, making it by far the most common practice. However, despite its popularity, it is not without some liabilities. The more waste put in a landfill, the more space it takes up, thus requiring more land to meet disposal demands. Given the resistance on the part of the public for new landfill construction near residential communities, this poses a problem.

Beyond the issues of the volume of trash and the space needed for disposal, the environment is also not immune to landfills. The decomposition process for buried waste releases gases into the atmosphere. The two most common of these are methane and carbon dioxide, both of which are greenhouse gases. These are not the only products of decomposition. Other gases are also released that cause the odors typically associated with trash and landfills. While these compounds are typically only given off in trace amounts, they have an affect on the local area, and a minor long term affect on the atmosphere and air quality. Since these substances are combustible, landfill gas is typically burned to produce energy by the generation of electricity (like incinerators), or to simply reduce environmental impact (Tammemagi 111-113).

Landfills also result in the production a hazardous liquid called leachate, which is formed when water from the outside environment and the decomposition process is mixed with the various substances in a landfill. Typically it contains many heavy metals, organic compounds and dissolved solids that can be hazardous in large quantities (Tammemagi 107-109). This liquid waste poses a particular threat because in older landfills that do not have liners (and in newer ones where they have failed), it seeps into the underlying soils and contaminates groundwater, which is the source of drinking water for local communities who have private wells instead of a public water supply.

Many argue that landfills are a safe, cheap and cost effective way to dispose of trash. While this is mostly very true, this argument tends to overlook the external or hidden costs associated with landfilling that have just been discussed. Though great care is taken to make landfills environmentally friendly and safe, they are imperfect means of disposal and ought to reflect their liabilities in the cost of disposing waste in them. These faults include permanent loss of land for other uses, damage to the atmosphere from gases and to groundwater from leachate (Tammemagi 38). While it may seem these flaws are catastrophic, the reality is their impact is not as substantial as many environmentalists advocate. Landfills are predominantly a safe and practical way to dispose of trash, and they continue to improve. However, their liabilites are an invitation to examining other methods of disposal.

One alternative to direct landfilling is incineration, which is the burning of trash at high temperature. According to the EPA web site of Solid Waste Basic Facts, this accounts for roughly fifteen percent of disposal in the United States. Often, the energy released from combustion is used to generate electricity. This practice is an effective means of getting a return on trash, but there are also environmental issues. As with any combustion facility, waste incinerators emit many gases out the stack based on what the burned material contains. Thus, modern incinerators that are properly maintained and constructed are much more expensive to operate, as they are required by law to clean these emissions gases before releasing them to prevent health and atmospheric problems (Porter 74-75).

Exhaust gas is not the only product of incineration. As with any fire, ash is also left behind. In this case, the ash is the same waste that was initially burned, and according to the EPA web site of Solid Waste Basic Facts, it is reduced ninety percent by volume and seventy-five percent by weight as a result of the gaseous products that escape during the combustion reaction. These facts may make incineration appear to be an excellent option. However, though the ash is greatly reduced from the initial trash volume, it still contains the same toxins that were in the initial waste, as these are not always consumed in combustion. As a result, these toxins are far more concentrated in the ash than the initial waste, making it more hazardous to deal with (Porter 75). Not only that, but incinerators can't keep ash forever. It must also be disposed of, and the best facilities for that are landfills. This links back to their function and impact as previously discussed because incineration involves disposal on two levels: first by burning, and second by landfilling the leftovers.

While incineration saves on the volume of trash that goes into landfills, it also contributes other pollutants. Recycling does the same, while not polluting near as much, and instead providing materials that may be returned to the production industry. In fact, recycling can be used to reduce the amount of material in the conventional waste stream before it even reaches landfills or incinerators. As of 2001 figures, the top waste substance is paper, (a recyclable product) at 35.7 percent of the total. The third largest waste materials are plastics, which constitute 11.1 percent of the total (Municipal 8). Not only are they recyclable, but also a non-renewable resource as they're produced from petroleum. Taking these items and others such as metal cans and glass bottles out of the waste stream by recycling lessens the amount of trash that would otherwise be disposed of in a landfill or incinerator. Reducing the sheer volume of garbage sent to these facilities slows the rate at which they are consumed, and lowers their impact.

Cost Analysis: Virgin Supplies, Recycling, and Programs

Virgin materials are the primary competitors with recycled products. This makes sense because they are the initial source of all recyclables, as they are extracted directly from the earth by mining, drilling, foresting, or other practices. In discussing these materials, it is necessary to briefly look at the impact their production has on the planet. Consider the production of virgin paper against the alternative practice of recycling. Allen Hershkowitz has said regarding this issue that "While modern paper recycling mills produce no hazardous wastes, the virgin pulp and paper industry is one of the world's largest generators of toxic air pollutants, surface water pollution, sludge, and solid wastes." Obtaining other virgin products is often not much better in practice. Ores that must be obtained by mining are not always easy to access. Not only that, but the Earth has limited resources in the ground, and the supply will one day be exhausted if care is not taken. Extraction also results in pollution by heavy machinery, and from substances causing hazardous water runoff (Hershkowitz). Finally, crude oil must not be overlooked, as it is one of the most consumed natural resources in the world today. Its uses extend far beyond running automobiles, heaters, ships and airplanes. Oil is also required in the production of plastic materials and asphalt concretes such as road pavements. Since the supply is limited and will one day be exhausted, alternatives to continued production through the use of virgin materials ought to be investigated.

Unfortunately, the prices of virgin materials and products typically don't reflect the external costs on the environment, the health of the public, or the availability of materials for the future. The prices also exclude many tax subsidies, typically adding to billions of dollars (Platt and Seldman). Therefore, virgin materials have a clear cost advantage over recycled products, which do not receive any of these breaks. Thus, the market for recycling is difficult, and involves a challenge on a monetary cost effectiveness basis.

Recycling saves on the environmental and public issues aspect of virgin production. Using recovered materials slows the exhaustion of certain non-renewable resources, and in some cases even reduces or eliminates the need for virgin materials production. Recycling also saves on the cost of the wasteful practice of disposing these materials in landfills. Even so, while it may seem like the perfect A+ solution the world needs, there still remain other factors to consider, most especially regarding the cost of the practice itself.

Municipalities that instituted recycling programs in the late 1980s and early 1990s were often not entirely prepared to pay the bill for the task they aggressively embarked upon. Mandatory recycling programs come at a high price. In fact, to keep them functional, there are enforcement costs to make sure everyone is participating properly, collection costs from the gathering of recyclable material separate from other waste, and there are processing costs for it at Material Recovery Facilities, known as MRFs. In these MRFs, recyclables are sorted through a variety of methods from mechanical to by hand, before being baled for later shipping to a plant that desires the material (Tammemagi 48-52). As a result of what's involved, this process can be very expensive. The more recyclables collected, the greater the cost to handle them because it is much more work to process them all from pickup through the MRFs. Some recyclable materials are also very difficult, expensive, or inefficient to recycle at this time because technology or current available methods are not practical (Porter 125-126). Thus, municipal programs demanding the recycling of such materials without careful planning first could be placing an unnecessary and large bill on their community budgets.

The most common argument against recycling is that it just plain costs too much, far more than other methods of disposal. This can be true in some cases, but typically, those who make this argument are really evaluating cost failure of a recycling program, not the practice itself. John Tierney does this in a very commonly referenced article titled "Recycling Is Garbage" when he says,

> The recycling program consumes resources. It requires extra administrators and a continual public relations campaign explaining what to do with dozens of different products—recycle milk jugs, but not milk cartons, index cards but not construction paper. (Most New Yorkers still don't know the rules.) It requires enforcement agents to inspect garbage and issue tickets. Most of all, it requires extra collection crews and trucks. Collecting a ton of recyclable items is three times more expensive than collecting a ton of garbage because the crews pick up less material at each stop. For every ton of glass, plastic and metal that the truck delivers to a private recycler, the city currently spends $200 more than it would spend to bury the material in a landfill.

In this evaluation of recycling, Tierney specifically references the program implemented in New York City, and the aspects where it fails to be cost effective, not the success or failure of recycling as a whole, which would involve all aspects and costs, both internal and external. Thus, while the New York program may make recycling seem to be nonsense, a judgment based on one failure should not be assumed to be global.

A similar argument based on cost is made by Christopher Douglass when he explains recycling programs processing items such as newsprint, magazines, aluminum cans, plastic, and glass, have an average collection cost of about $139 a ton. He then goes on to explain an average of an additional $86 a ton goes into MRF operation and proper sorting, while the savings from not using landfills for the disposal of these materials are only about $27 a ton. Hence, the total cost of collecting and processing recyclables in the average program is about $198 for every ton disposed (Douglass). While this is a much more accurate painting of recycling programs in their entirety, nowhere does the argument account for the income from the sale of recycled materials back to manufacturing industries, which can play a substantial role in offsetting the cost of running recycling programs.

Recycling in Context of Other Current Practices— What's Effective?

In order for the recycling practice to be viable and cost effective, sound municipal and community programs must be implemented in place of those that are struggling. These should include a detailed plan for recycling and a thorough cost analysis in order to prevent situations like the economic problems in New York pointed out by Tierney. Based on observation and evaluation, the best recycling programs are those that have involved incremental and transformative changes. These have the greatest overall outcomes economically and ecologically (Weinberg, Pellow and Schnaiberg 150). It's better to have a strategy and a long term goal than to rush into overnight changes and demand for recycling all reusable materials at once. Such practice causes a type of overload on the system, and is nearly impossible to implement.

Substantial costs due to the expenses of recycling should be limited. As previously mentioned, when current recycling practices are inefficient or under-developed, landfilling is still a good option (Porter 125-126). Though there are drawbacks and certain issues to disposing waste in them as discussed, overall they are one of the safest and best methods currently in existence for solid waste disposal. Thus, instead of focusing on attempting to recover and recycle all possible materials, the most efficient practices available should be used for cost effectiveness. Communities should recycle items such that the resale value of the material cancels the net cost of actually doing the recycling, or even makes a profit (Porter 141). Also, the costs/prices should balance between virgin production and recycling practices to allow for optimum savings and economic benefits. The supply and demand system will ultimately work in favor of recycling, as virgin materials become less accessible and more expensive, recycling old material will become the cheaper option, and the market for it will grow as the playing field is leveled between these two options. Those items currently not able to be recycled such that cost and resale values balance should be disposed as regular waste. New procedures actually do allow for later access.

Landfills can now be mined to extract materials from them that were once disposed as waste. This process can reclaim recyclable materials once thrown away in them at a later date, when it is much more economical or necessary based on demand to recycle them (Porter 125). This practice does have costs associated with it, but the benefits are more than just reclaiming once disposed recyclable materials. Mining landfills also removes items from them, thus reducing the volume of trash, which allows for the disposal of more solid waste and can reduce environmental impact (Porter 125, Tammemagi, 130).

It may seem that the argument has now turned on recycling. This is not the case. While recycling is a genuinely good practice, its implementation often tends to fail. Citizens ought to recognize this and embrace the practice if they are truly being good stewards of the world and its resources, while at the same time work for cost effectiveness. Currently, procedures should be a matter of what's wise and realistic based on the engrained practices of society and industry. Expecting to be able to recycle all possible materials cost effectively overnight is absurd, but that is what many have tried to do. Instead of one giant leap, small steps should be taken to slowly move toward the ultimate goal of recycling and reuse in order to bring about transformation in the waste disposal system. Hence the responsibility lies on everyone for assured success and future development.

Conclusion

Overall, recycling of municipal solid waste is a good practice. It's important to realize that there are no instant results or gratification for implementing it. Instead, these lie in the future as recycling saves the environment by reducing trash disposal in landfills and incinerators and wastefulness on the part of society. Though recycling everything now is not viable, looking to the future does require starting now, such that programs can be established and developed by the time they are absolutely necessary. Recycling may produce initial costs, but these are small when future ramifications to the environment and society are considered. Citizens should recycle, and continue to do so according to local regulations and requirements, possibly even working toward continued program development and effectiveness. While the benefits may not be clear now, those generations to come will appreciate them.

Works Cited

Ackerman, Frank. *Why Do We Recycle?*. Washington, DC: Island Press, 1997.

Douglass, Christopher. "Recycling Programs Are Unprofitable and Unnecessary." *Government's Hand in the Recycling Market: A New Decade* (1998). *Current Controversies*. Thomson Gale. University of New Hampshire, Dimond Lib., Durham, NH. 9 November 2004 <http://galenet.galegroup.com>.

Hershkowitz, Allen. "Recycled Materials Produce Less Pollution." Social Research (1998). *Current Controversies.* Thomson Gale. University of New Hampshire, Dimond Lib., Durham, NH. 9 November 2004 <http://galenet.galegroup.com>.

Municipal Solid Waste in the United States: 2001 Facts and Figures Executive Summary. Nov. 2003. 29 October 2004 <http://www.epa.gov/ epaoswer/non-hw/muncpl/pubs/msw-sum01.pdf>.

Platt, Brenda and Neil Seldman. "Efficient Recycling Programs Can Reduce Waste." From the Ground Up June/July 2000. *Current Controversies.* Thomson Gale. University of New Hampshire, Dimond Lib., Durham, NH. 9 November 2004 <http://galenet.galegroup.com>.

Porter, Richard C. *The Economics of Waste.* Washington, DC: Resources for the Future, 2002.

Tammemagi, Hans. *The Waste Crisis Landfills, Incinerators, and the Search for a Sustainable Future.* New York: Oxford University Press, 1999.

Tierney, John. "Recycling is Garbage." *The New York Times* 30 June 1996, late edition. Lexis Nexis. University of New Hampshire, Dimond Lib., Durham, NH. 15 November 2004 <http://web.lexis-nexis.com>.

United States. Environmental Protection Agency. *Municipal Solid Waste: Basic Facts.* 27 April 2004. 29 October 2004 <http://www.epa.gov/ epapswer/non-hw/muncpl/facts.htm>.

Weinberg, Adam S., David N. Pellow, and Allen Schnaiberg. *Urban Recycling and the Search for Sustainable Community Development.* Princeton: Princeton University Press, 2000.

Works Consulted

Hershkowitz, Allen. "Recycling Is an Effective Means of Preventing Solid Waste Pollution." *San Diego Union-Tribune.* 21 Sept. 1997. *Current Controversies.* Thomson Gale. University of New Hampshire, Dimond Lib., Durham, NH. 9 November 2004 http://galenet.galegroup.com>.

Leroux, Kivi. "Recycling's War of Words." *Waste Age.* 1 April 2000. 29 October 2004 <http://wasteage.com/mag/waste_recyclings_war_words/index.html>.

Section 2

Student Writing
from across the Disciplines

A Classroom of Fairness

19

Meredith A. Bailey

Zoology 690 Evolution
for the assignment see chapter 24
for the writing guide see chapter 30

One of the founding principles of the United States is the ideal of equal rights for all and the preventing of trivialization of any views, minority or otherwise. To some, this means that the religious dogma known as "Creation Science" has a valid stance within the public school science classroom alongside the scientifically-accepted theory of evolution. Creationism, anti-evolutionists claim, is a valid explanation for the origin of life and as such deserves "equal treatment" in the classroom, being presented as a scholastically-endorsed alternative to evolution. This, claim Creationists, is only fair. But is it really? Or are Creationists simply bent on forcing their religious ideologies on a captive audience of schoolchildren under the guise of valid scientific knowledge?

Creationists feel that it is "unfair for science to exclude supernatural explanations" particularly in the education of children; that is, those who will become the scientists of the next generation (Lovell 2002). This, right from the beginning, highlights one of the fallacies of the Creationist standpoint: science studies the natural world, not the supernatural. Science is concerned with astronomy, not astrology; chemistry, not alchemy; medicine, not voodoo witchcraft. Authentic science has for centuries been "excluding supernatural explanations" for naturally-occurring phenomenon on the grounds that the universe behaves according to certain inherent physical and chemical properties based on atomic structure and interactions of simple and complex molecules—not because God simply feels like making the sun rise in the east (Matsumura 2001). True scientific theories do not rely on miracles, as Creationism does, nor do they assume exceptions to the physical properties of the universe.

In many state school systems, science education concerning evolution has already suffered at the hands of the anti-evolutionists so it can hardly be said that evolution itself is receiving "fair" treatment. States have avoided writing curriculum standards involving evolution, or even containing the word, in an attempt to avoid controversy. In Ohio, for example, statewide standards on the teaching of evolution were still nonexistent in 2000, and public school curricula frequently replaced "evolution," with "change over time," effectively marginalizing evolutionary theory, and not fully recognizing or representing evolution as the valid scientific natural force that it is (Evans 2002). Worse, some states permit the teaching of evolutionary theory, but with the stipulation that it be accompanied by the detracting publishing of a disclaimer, dismissing evolution as merely a "theory" (Meikle 2001). Since 1995, Alabama has mandated a disclaimer on evolution be pasted into state-approved science texts. This disclaimer was expanded in 2001 from a one-paragraph description of evolution as an "unproved belief" to a four-paragraph injunction to students to "learn to make distinctions between the multiple meanings of evolution" and to keep an "open mind" (Meikle 2001). The request to "keep an open mind" was likewise part of the original 1995 evolution disclaimer, and appears frequently in arguments in support of Creationism—for indeed, one does need an open mind to ignore empirical scientific evidence and subscribe to views attributing all functioning of the natural world to supernatural forces.

Clinging to scientifically-supported theories, such as evolution, and presenting them as such in a science classroom is, to a Creationist, closed-minded and unfair. An anti-evolution bill introduced in the state of Washington finds "the teaching of the theory of evolution in the common schools of the state of Washington is repugnant to the principles of the Declaration of Independence and thereby unconstitutional and unlawful," and calls for the replacement of all textbooks that present evolution with textbooks that "teach the self-evident truth of creation" (Updates 2002). This unreasonable bill, which was defeated, does not even attempt the illusion of "fairness" that Creationists generally endorse and attempt to infiltrate into legitimate science disciplines.

Creationists are frequently unfair themselves as they pursue their quest to insert their ideologies into the science classroom. In their efforts to force Creationism on public school science classes, anti-evolutionists tend to misrepresent themselves: an Intelligent Design advocacy group in Ohio has dubbed themselves "Science Excellence for All Ohioans," carefully distancing themselves both from the directed-descent dogma they embrace as well as the evolutionary theory they oppose. The propagandic result of this causes those who oppose Intelligent Design to be viewed as opposed to excellence in science, or against education altogether (Evans 2002). Intelligent Design advocates are equally eager to distance themselves from conventional young-earth creationists, citing lack of religion or specified designer in their ideology. But even here they misrepresent themselves with beautifully muddied logic: the Intelligent Design dogma only makes an *inference* of a higher power acting as a designer. Because they use similarly fuzzy terminology in description of their ideas and avoid a specification of that designer, they are not referring to a god, and hence, not to religion; thus, their philosophy is a valid scientific viewpoint (Evans 2002). However, both the public at large and the scientific community regard Intelligent Design as "creationism in a cheap tuxedo" (Evans 2002). Creationists, crying for fairness, are treating evolution as unfairly as they feel they are themselves being treated. Many of the changes that Creationists propose or attempt to bring into the classroom are designed specifically to undermine evolution in a sort of character attack. These include putting lengthy disclaimers in textbooks, as in Alabama; placing Creationist theologians alongside legitimate scientists, and, perhaps worst of all, actually removing factual evidence and information from biology books, such as the scientifically-determined and accepted age of the earth and the universe. Creationists attempting to put holes in evolutionary theory have cited as evidence the gaps in Charles Darwin's illustration of the divergence of taxa from *On the Origin of Species*. They claim it endeavors—and fails—to present the origin of major animal groups, which was not the illustration's intent, further displaying Creationists' inability or unwillingness to learn or use the resources needed to have a meaningful, educational discussion concerning evolution (Miller 2002).

Creationists further misrepresent, through ignorance or through intent, the basic scientific terminology that is critical to comprehension of evolution. This inability to correctly use or understand the biological vocabulary fundamental to the discussion severely undermines the Creationist standpoint even as they are attempting to refute evolution, dismissing it as merely theory. Creationists use the word *theory* in the popular sense of the word: a speculation that is subject to an equal amount of doubt and credibility. In the scientific definition of the word, as with the theory of evolution, *theory* refers to an established and accepted explanation used to describe a set of observations verifiable by repetition. A theory, in the scientific sense, is for all intents and purposes, *true*—or, true in-so-far as there has not yet been substantial evidence to significantly counter, dispute or overturn it. Atomic theory, Einstein's Theory of Relativity, and

Newton's Theory of Gravity are not any less true because they are theories. The important distinction between evolutionary theory and Creationist theory is that evolution is based on years of quantified, replicable and scientifically-verifiable observation and experimentation, whereas Creationism is based on a varied collection of legends that were initially recorded 2,000 years ago, and probably after considerable alteration due to previous oral relation.

While Creationists opine that presenting only evolution in the classroom is unfair, they do not stop to consider what the forced imposition of Creation Science on the average schoolchild will do to that student's perceptions of how the scientific method is used. For example, young-earth Creationists, in direct disregard for proven techniques for age estimation, such as isotope dating (which, incidentally, was used to accurately date the Dead Sea Scrolls, the earliest Biblical writings), believe that the earth is several thousand to a few million years old rather than the 4 to 5 billion years old geologists and other scientists have estimated it to be (Scrolls 2002). Some Young-earth Creationists, as a result of this belief, even desire references to the earth's age be stricken from biology textbooks (Evans 2002). This does not teach science to schoolchildren; this teaches rather that when scientific evidence conflicts with one's personal opinions, it is perfectly acceptable and academically valid to dismiss scientific fact in preference for one's own beliefs. This lesson is the exact antithesis of how scientific evaluation and experimentation is supposed to function. Students who continue in the science field while retaining this erroneous idea are probably doomed to a short career in their chosen discipline, and it is certainly unfair of Creationists to allow their religious dogmas to set up students for failure.

Some students are perceptive enough to see through the Creationist deception and are courageous enough to respond. "The intent of this disclaimer" wrote one Alabama student in a newspaper editorial in response to the state's expanded evolution disclaimer, "is to discourage teachers from teaching evolution—the basis for all biology. This is roughly equivalent to teaching chemistry by saying "No one has seen atoms, so their existence remains controversial" (Collins 2001). With Creationists enforcing sub-standard scientific education on not only their own children but on others' pupils as well, they are jeopardizing the future educations of these students. "I can see myself sitting down with the admissions committee," continues this same Alabama high-school student, "and worrying whether they are thinking, "Oh, this is that kid from Alabama, where the school board mandates seventeenth century biology" (Collins 2001). By attempting to force unscientific, theology-based conjectures into the public school classrooms, Creationists are pushing students away from learning and, for those driven individuals who yet retain a desire for an education still grounded in reality and science, Alabama Creationists are pushing them out of the state. Students who are too perceptive to be taken in by the vocal Creationists' claptrap will join the "brain drain" and leave the "seventeenth century biology" of Alabama behind them in their search for quality science education (Collins 2001). Creationists are unable to see that their insistence on forcing religion into the science classroom is only hurting themselves and their own state.

But one question that has not yet arisen in the majority of the Creationism in the classroom debates revolves around the qualifications of science teachers to provide a Creationist history of the natural world. When anti-evolution education standards were a proposed addition to Hawaii's science curriculum, religious leaders surprisingly spoke out alongside the evolutionists in rejection of the new Creationist curriculum, firmly stating their opposition to state science teachers taking on the roles of religious educators (Pyle 2000). To be strictly "fair," if Creationism is taught in a science classroom, then religious educators should spend an equal amount of time presenting evolution in their Sunday School classes. However, just like the qualifications of science teachers presenting religion may be called into question, the ability of most people untrained in science education—as a religious figure is likely to be—to accurately present and discuss the intricacies and ramifications of evolutionary theory is variable or questionable at best. What happens when a Buddhist or Hindu science teacher is called upon to present Christian theology in a science classroom? It is entirely possible that a teacher put in this position is not only unqualified to teach the ideology of Creationist Science, but may feel a distinct degree of resentment at being forced to do so in preference to their own religious beliefs. Even within Christianity, the religious basis for Creation Science, the diversity of religious sects provides ample scope for a variety of interpretations of the Genesis legend, and the division between those with Protestant viewpoints and those holding to Catholicism can be as sharp as those between Christianity and Islam. Furthermore, Native American nations have always held the status of sovereign nations within the United States under constitutional law. Will they, too, be forced to present Christian theology under the guise of science to their students and told that this is fair?

Creationists are incredibly concerned about presenting both sides of the issue in the classroom, but they do not seem to consider that there are more than two sides to this issue. If Christian theology is presented as scientific fact alongside evolution in a science classroom, is a Hindu or

Jewish student supposed to accept that without question? The Creationists do not seem to care that they are trivializing other conceivable origins and religions in their mission to force their dogma onto school biology curricula. If Genesis is a recognizable alternative to evolution, then the Classical mythology of Prometheus is a valid explanation for why man is able to use fire. Likewise, the Iroquois creation legend of Sky-Woman falling from the clouds to land on the back of a giant turtle should be taught in the biology classroom, along with the similar Norse myth of the giantess falling to earth from her cold palace, as well as the creation stories of the Inuit, Chinese, Navajo, Buddhist and every other religion and nationality on earth. The difficulty with this sort of equal treatment of alternatives to evolution—which, if Creationists succeed in pushing into the science class, *should* be fully implemented—is that it engenders no longer a biology class, but a class in comparative religion.

Creationists further object that by denying the divinity of human creation, evolutionary theory is detrimental to basic morality. But can there not be codes of morality—that is, a basic sense of decency—that is not derived from religion? This objection often raised by Creationists is a *non sequitur* to the real argument: for what school has "morality education" as a part of its stated curriculum? The goal of a teacher is to present information, not to instill in students their own beliefs on morality, something children, by the age they start school, should already have a very firm handle on from their parents, guardians, or other sources. Moral instruction and science education are two very different worlds, and should be treated as such. Religion attempts to address and control both of these fields, and often to combine them by reducing them to useless simplicity. It is a disservice to both morality and science to lump them together under the guise of being one and the same thing. Furthermore, there is equal argument that evolution reinforces morality, rather than undermines it, as the Creationists claim: "Understanding evolution reinforces the message that all people are important parts of the web of life, and each person is unique and valuable" (Matsumura 2001). Under evolution, this can be expanded to say rather that "each *organism* is unique and valuable," an acknowledgement that the Bible, with its messages to overtake and subjugate the earth, does not make.

Individuals outside of the scientific community have, in general, an illusion that science is in pursuit of the truth, and that this is the sole goal and reason for its existence. This is a poor assessment of the science profession, which is instead on a quest for *understanding*. Biologists, like other scientists, know the "personal satisfaction in *figuring things out*" (Pond 2002). The field of science, and still more that of biology, is in a constant state of flux, partly because it involves the study of living, dynamic systems. The best we can hope for is an understanding—that is, our perception of what is true at one given point in time and space—before an alteration in this dynamic system alters our perceptions of it again. In many cases, these changes happen in predictable, naturally-occurring patterns, but not always. This makes for a potent argument against Intelligent Design and other Creationist rhetoric: If some unmanifested supernatural higher power were really in control, there would be no deviation from the norm—every biological event would be identical to all others before. Since there would be no chance, as occurs with natural selection and evolution, there would be no need for change and variation, and all systems would become immediately fixed and static, a contingency almost completely removed from the realm of possibility. In fact I have, in using "almost," just exemplified the inability of science to state ideas as *true*. Yet it is accepted and understood that the possibility of all systems becoming fixed and unchanging, as would happen under an intelligent designer, is so close to zero as to be essentially nil. If science were really about finding truth, the haziness surrounding the popular and the scientific definitions of words like *theory* would not exist. Theories are the scientific equivalents of truths, a distinction Creationists proponents fail to understand when they dismiss evolution as merely a theory.

Those citing fairness are likewise missing a very important reality: life is *not* fair, inside or outside of the realm of biology. Natural selection acts to weed out those least fit for survival; thus from life's outset some individuals have advantages over others which makes them more suited for survival. If life were fair, then each individual would have an equal chance for survival with all others of their kind, generating the same sort of homogeneity as an Intelligent Designer described above. Creationists also fail to confront the fossil record and extinction—would not an Intelligent Designer, or God, being infallible, have created perfect creatures capable of infinite resourcefulness and unsupported hypothesis that these certain inequities God purposefully placed in these organisms—in which case, is no God arbitrarily earmarking specific individuals for hardship, suffering, and death, or even complete extinction? And is this not the very definition of unfair? So callous and inhumane a deity might well deserve to have no faith placed in him. Natural selection is at least based on chance, and randomness can hardly be accused of being biased. The fairness of chance drives natural selection and evolution, and the adaptive advantages generated by these forces create the unfairness that is life. Natural selection applies to more than animals, however: pseudo-scientific theories like

Creationism can be driven to extinction, allowing the more fit explanation of evolution to endure.

Works Cited

Collins, Luke. "A Student Responds to the Alabama Disclaimer." *Reports of the National Center for Science Education.* Vol 21, No. 3-4, May-Aug, 2001.

Edwords, Frederick. "Is it Really Fair to Give Creationism Equal Time?" *Scientists Confront Creationism.* Ed. Laurie R. Godfrey. W.W. Norton & CO, 1983, New York.

Evans, Skip. "Ohio: The Next Kansas?" *Reports of the National Center for Science Education.* Vol. 22, No. 1-2, Jan/Apr 2002.

Lovell, Frank. "Ohio Forum: Why ID is not Science." *Reports of the National Center for Science Education.* Vol. 22, No. 1-2, Jan/Apr 2002.

Matsumura, Molleen. "Evolution, Creation, and Science Education: Answers to Ten Common Questions." *Reports of the National Center for Science Education.* Vol. 21, No. 3-4, May-Aug, 2001.

Meikle, Eric. "Alabama Upgrades Disclaimer." *Reports of the National Center for Science Education.* Vol. 21, No. 3-4, May-Aug, 2001.

Miller, Kenneth R. "Goodbye, Columbus." *Reports of the National Center for Science Education.* Vol. 22, No. 1-2, Jan/Apr 2002.

Pond, Jean. "Science and Christianity: What's Wrong with Creationism and "Intelligent Design?" *Reports of the National Center for Science Education.* Vol. 22, No. 1-2, Jan/Apr 2002.

Pyle, Richard. "Anti-Evolution Standards Rejected in Hawaii." *Reports of the National Center for Science Education.* Vol. 20, No. 6, Nov/Dec 2000.

"Scrolls from the Dead Sea: The Ancient Library of Qumran and Modern Scholarship." Library of Congress, February 27, 2002. http://lcweb.loc.gov/exhibits/scrolls/

"Updates: Washington." *Reports of the National Center for Science Education.* Vol. 22, No. 1-2, Jan/Apr 2002.

20

Part the Waters with MOSES: Working to Revolutionize Water Skiing

Steff Kelsey and Greg Wolff

Mechanical Engineering 755: Senior Design Project I

Executive Summary

When characterizing a top of the line waterski, the same key features are always highlighted. Slalom waterskis must have a great acceleration, a smooth turn, a large holding angle, and a huge deceleration. Waterski manufacturers have been struggling with design tradeoffs in order to maximize each ski's performance. Likewise, elite skiers have been utilizing the cutting edge in training in order to set new records in this young and exciting sport.

The *MOSES* automated wing system is targeted toward the training of slalom waterskiers. With the aid of push-button wing control, skiers will be able to negotiate slalom courses at world record rope lengths. Successfully completing a world record course would give the skier the "feel" for the type of acceleration and deceleration needed to compete at the world-class level. The concept for the *MOSES* system was derived from the physical and biomechanics of present day slalom skiers. Design work was done from breaking down the essential physics of negotiating a slalom course as well the fluid dynamics of the water around the ski to drafting up concepts using CAD systems.

The *MOSES* system consists of a rotating wing driven by a high speed, high torque remote control servo. The servo is controlled by a two-channel 75mHz AM receiver. The receiver accepts signal from a two-channel transmitter. The mechanical system is built from stock aluminum. The entire system is simple and light, a try efficient design.

The *MOSES* system was verified utilizing a four phase test process. The first phase was designed to create data curves relating wing angle to overall drag on the ski with the wing fixed at known angles at 8.2 mph and again at 30 mph. These curves could then be compared to curves generated from drag data taken while the *MOSES* system rotates the wing in high velocity flows. A favorable comparison of the curves would verify the design. A comprehensive test was also planned where the system would be tested with a skier onboard in order to measure the change in acceleration and deceleration in an actual slalom course as well as giving the "feel" of the system; that unquantifiable number that is the true measure of performance in sports products.

The *MOSES* system did very well at low velocities, but the test plan was greatly flawed at high velocities leading to inconclusive results. More work must be done before *MOSES* can be brought to the level of comprehensive testing and the objectives truly met.

Introduction

> ". . . every single one of the characteristics you should expect out of an elite ski; phenomenal acceleration, a smooth predictable turn, gargantuan angle, ability to hold that angle, and unsurpassed deceleration."
> —2002 Connelly F1 press release

Background

When marketing tournament series waterskis, major ski companies always plug the same characteristics. Elite skiers demand stability while turning at high speeds, rapid deceleration before the turn, and rapid acceleration out of the turn. Every ski company has their own innovation to attacking the demands on performance. Conelly and O'Brien, the two leading manufacturers, both claim to have adjusted the rocker, the balance point of the ski between the tip and the tail, and the flex so that the acceleration and deceleration characteristics of the ski are maximizing performance.

Why are world-class skiers concerned with these characteristics? It comes down to the course that they have to negotiate. Skiers must round six buoys, 37.5 feet from the center of the boat, at the shortest possible rope length. In order to travel the path at shorter rope lengths, the velocity of the skier between the buoys must be more than double that of the ski-boat. Naturally, a skier attempting a sharp slalom turn at speeds in excess of seventy miles per hour will end up cart-wheeling across the water. The skier must decelerate quickly before each buoy, yet accelerate immediately after turning to keep up with the speeding boat.

In order for a skier to slow down before a turn on any tournament water ski, he or she must rock forward, increasing the wetted surface areas of the underbelly of the ski as well as decreasing the negative angle of attack of the wing. A larger negative wing angle increases the projected wing surface area in the plane normal to velocity and increases drag. In order to maximize acceleration out of a turn, the skier must do the opposite and lean back, decreasing the wetted-surface area of the underbelly and decreasing the projected surface area of the wing, reducing overall draft. Varying the wing shape changes the drag characteristics of the ski in these two phases, but always in a trade-off manner. Manufacturers can choose to shape the wing to either increase the acceleration phase or the deceleration phase, but never both.

Objectives

Team *MOSES* sought to give the skier direct control over the angle of the wing, thus giving more control of the acceleration and deceleration capabilities of the ski and improving waterski performance. The project was broken down into the following phases: design, fabrication, verification.

The objective of the design phase was to turn ideas into dimensional realities. Team *MOSES* brainstormed different possibilities for giving the skier more control in a slalom course and then give various concepts a trial by rigorous fluid dynamics analysis in the hope of selecting the most efficient concept in terms of cost, function, and durability.

The objective of the fabrication phase was to make the dimensioned concepts into working systems and subsystems. The fabrication phase held the greatest dangers for the budge and was fraught with the most tense moments of the project. Dimensioned drawings are often a long way off from what can actually be machined.

The verification phase was implemented to compare the functions of the completed prototype with those of the design phase. Team *MOSES* specifically needed to find if the wing angle was being changed at various speeds, changing the drag characteristics of the ski at the push of a button. The ultimate objective was to find that *MOSES* system worked at speeds comparable to those used by elite skier in a slalom course as well as still "feeling" great within the course, as in the added systems do not detract from the pre-existing performance of the waterski.

Approach

Design

The objective was to improve the performance of a waterski. Team *MOSES* elected to attack this objective by focusing on the fin and wing assembly of a slalom ski. The design process began by finding the dimensions of a typical slalom ski wing and fin assembly. Second, a fluids analysis was applied so that forces on the wing could be found at different angles and varying speeds. Possible drag forces gave information regarding the change in ski character with varying wing angle, while changes in lift gave an idea of what force would be necessary in order to change the wing angle while skiing at different velocities.

With the data, team *MOSES* was able to move into servo selection. Remote control servos come in a variety of shapes and sizes, are easy stock parts to implement, and are relatively cheap when compared to the labor and headache of fabricating digital potential controllers in-house. Team *MOSES* chose a servo from Futaba, an internationally known manufacturer of remote control parts. The S5302 marine servo was selected for having high speed and high torque capabilities. The S5302 pushes an incredible 236 oz/in (24.75 lb/in) of torque at the speed of 60 degrees per 0.15 seconds while weighing only 4.4 ounces. The servo fit in nicely under the force requirement curves and in the dimensional constraints.

Next, the linkage between servo and the wing was analyzed for strength under the maximum possible speed conditions.

Construction

After parts were acquired over winter break and over the month of February, the true fabrication of the *MOSES* system began. Fortunately, the design is simple and small, requiring few materials. Unfortunately, being small, the parts were often hard to work with for amateur machinists. The approach was as follows.

The first attack in the machine shop was to mount the servo onto the designated fin and wing assembly. A u-clamp was machined, thanks to the genius of Bob Champlin, and the servo was fixed to the topside of the fin. Next, a slot was machined from the rear wing mounting hole to the top of the fin (the clearance for the servo linkage). A linkage arm was found among stock remote control parts that was only ⅛" in diameter, pre-curved to fit any servo arm, and pre-threaded to link to any tapped part. Using this stock part, the *MOSES* team made a tiny mounting bracket with a ⅛" tap on the top and hole fitting the wing screw across the lower wide. A bit of machining to the stock wings and the *MOSES* system was almost ready for action.

The second to last step in the process was mounting the RC parts. The parts were to be contained in a waterproof chamber. They were fitted with Velcro to secure them inside the chamber yet leaving them easily removable, an asset during the testing phases.

The last phase was fabricating a waterproof chamber for the RC parts and for the servo. The RC parts were placed in a modified piece of kitchen Tupperware. The Tupperware was mounted over some rubber, marine glue sealing the screw holes, and then secured with hiking straps to guard from physical damage. The servo was waterproofed with a ziplock bag, also easily removable, which had to be replaced between each test due to leakage. It remained effective for all testing phases.

Test and Evaluation

The test plan had four distinct phases. The first phase in the pan was indoor and outdoor drag testing with a fixed wing. The second phase was waterproof testing. The third phase indoor and outdoor drag testing with the *MOSES* system installed. The fourth and final phase was a comprehensive test.

The purpose of the fixed wing drag testing was to compile a curve of wing angle versus overall drag that can be used as basis for comparison when the *MOSES* system is activated and the drag re-tested in phase 3. The first phase was broken into two parts, the indoor and outdoor testing. The indoor test was performed at the Jere A. Chase Ocean Engineering Laboratory. The slalom ski was fixed to the Two Tank bracket and pushed, at 8.2 mpg, the length of the tank. The test was performed three times at each different wing angle (−5 to −30 degrees). The outdoor test was set to utilize a similar setup except gather data at 30 mph. Curves could then be drawn for wing angle versus overall ski drag.

The waterproof test was implemented at this point to ensure that all completed *MOSES* systems could be immersed in water with no damage to the delicate onboard electronics. The test consisted of dunking waterproof compartments in water and then checking the inside for moisture upon removal.

The purpose of phase 3 was to test *MOSES* systems on the setup from the first phase. The system was to be activated and placed in the indoor tow tank. During the run, instead of taking data from a fixed wing-ski, data would be taken as *MOSES* was rotating the wing. Drag curves generated from this phases could be compared to the phase one curves and evaluations made. The outdoor test was to be utilized in the same manner. The curve comparisons from this phase and the first phase would lend a strong indication as to the extent at which the *MOSES* system changed drag character of the ski.

The final testing phase, the comprehensive test, was to be the most telling in terms of actual ski performance. Roughly, the test consisted of setting up a digital camera and filming a skier executing a series of similar turns (as in a slalom course). The skier would negotiate the course without the aid of the *MOSES* system. The digital video camera, from a fixed position in the ski-boat, would record the skier's position as well as the portion of a marked section of the ski rope. Similar triangles could be used to find the skier's acceleration and deceleration orthogonal to the velocity vector of the ski craft. The test would be repeated, this time with the *MOSES* system at the fingertips of the skier. Deceleration and acceleration data in the plane normal to boat velocity *MOSES* and sin-*MOSES* could be compared. Also and most importantly, the skier could describe the "feel" of the *MOSES* system, which is a difficult variable to quantify when testing sports products for performance but is the real key to measuring success.

Description

The system is broken down into two main sub-systems: the handle and the fin and wing assembly. Connecting those two systems is the remote control equipment. Looking first at the triggering system for the device, a waterski handle was intended to house the transmitting device for the actuator, but the final design did not make it to that point. Size constraints and lack of spare parts combined with an unshakable fear of breaking the only working transmitter left team *MOSES* with the standard RC transmitter, one channel being used for the *MOSES* system.

The RC components that bridged that transmitter and the fin and wing assembly consist of the transmitter, a small receiver, a speed control with a power switch that served as a connection for the power source, a 7.2 volt NiCad battery, and the high speed/high torque servo.

The mechanical system consists of the servo, the linkage, the wing, and the altered fin. The servo is the Futaba S5302 high speed/high torque water-resistant marine model. The linkage is a two-piece system, the first being a one-eighth inch diameter armature that fits into the servo head and is threaded on the tail end. The threads fit into the second piece, a custom bracket that clasps a screw pin at the rear of the wing. The wing is pinned in two places by Phillips style screws. The fin has been hollowed out around the rear of the wing, a channel running the length of the fin from the rear wing pin to the servo base, all clearance for the armature. The fin is bolted to a slalom ski, the Connelly FX shaped hybrid; a midlevel slalom ski.

The *MOSES* system was altered for indoor and outdoor test phases. Both tests required an alternative mounting to the stock slalom bindings. A mounting bracket was machined from aluminum stock to fit the same screw pattern as the front binding. In the two tank test, the bracket was screwed directly into a force transducer using a ¼" x 28 x 1" stud. The force transducer was connected to the Jere A. Chase wireless LAN 2.4 Ghz data acquisition system.

The outdoor system consisted of the same bracket attached to the ski, except a rope around the bracket. Instead of the transducer being directly screwed into place, it was attached to the rope that tethered the ski to the boat, measuring the tension. The transducer was also wired into a strain indicator in a full Wheatstone bridge. The indicator was run into an AD port in a laptop computer that housed oscilloscope software.

Design Verification

The prototype was designed and fabricated with the intent of improving waterski performance. The test plan for verifying the performance of the *MOSES* system was broken into distinct phases, each with its own objective. The phases were as follows: Indoor drag test, outdoor drag test, waterproof test, indoor servo test, and comprehensive test.

The indoor drag test was designed to verify that the indoor tow tank apparatus was capable of collecting drag data. The apparatus consisted of the tow tank, the carriage extension, the ski clamp, the load cell, and the wireless LAN data collection system. The tow tank was simply a long slender pool with a carriage that straddled the pool. The carriage rode on a set of rails along the rim of the pool, a cable running the length of the tank wound around an AC pulled the carriage at a constant rate. The carriage extension was an approximately 3-foot length of aluminum channel stock that was clamped to the carriages so that it rode approximately 1.5 inches above the surface of the water. A hole was drilled in the channel stock at 2.5 inches above the water's surface. This was where the load cell attached the water ski to the carriage assembly.

The ski clamp consisted of a small section of 6-inch aluminum channel stock with two parallel threaded rods running through both walls of the channel stock. An aluminum plate was mounted on the two threaded rods and held in place with four nuts. This allowed the plate to be moved parallel to the ski to attach the ski at roughly its hydrodynamic center. The plate had a hole drilled at 2.5 inches above the surface of the water where the load cell was attached. The boot system was removed from the ski, and the ski clamp was attached using the screw holes as the boot system.

The load cell, a 25lbf Interface force transducer, was placed in a plastic bag and attached to the ski clamp using a ¼" x 28 x ¾" machine screw. The remaining end of the load cell was attached to the carriage extension using a ¼" x 28 x 1" stud. The data acquisition system included a strain indication, 12 volt DC power supply, an analog to digital converter, and a wireless digital transmitter. The data was collected by a digital receiver and recorded on a local computer. The recorded data was exported to Microsoft Excel files and analyzed. The load cell was calibrated.

The indoor test proceeded with the wing angle being fixed at −5 degrees and a run being performed. The speed of the carriage was set to 60 Hz. The computer was set to take data at 10 Hz for 12 seconds. This allows time for the experimenter to start collecting data and then start the carriage run. The data collection was started, and within two seconds the carriage run was begun. The carriage was run for the entire length of the tow tank. Once the data collection ceased, the acquired results were plotted. the data was trimmed so only the data on the plot corresponding to the forward movement of the carriage remained. This data was exported to an Excel file to be analyzed later. Three runs were performed at each angle of attack. The above procedure was repeated for 5 degree increments on the angle of attack of the wing to −35 degrees.

The collected data was compiled into a spreadsheet and analyzed. Since there was significant noise in the data, the average was taken over the period where the carriage was moving forward for each run. These results were scrutinized to be sure that they were consistent. Then the results for each angle of attack were averaged to have a final voltage representing the angle of attack. This final voltage was then converted to pounds of force using the calibration curve acquired earlier.

The raw data was characterized by heavy noise. In some cases there were spikes that exceeded the average value of data. This noise was the result of twisting of the carriage extension while holding the ski on the water during the run. Since channel lock is soft aluminum, it took a surprisingly small moment to cause the elastic twisting deformation. The noise was highly periodic, so it was averaged to find the mean value. It was originally thought to be possible to filter out the noise by using a simple Fourier transform. However the noise appeared to occur at roughly the same frequency as the data sample rate. Since the Fourier transform required a sample rate of at least twice the desired frequency to be captured, this method was not implemented. The average of the recorded values centered noise; the magnitude of the noise in both the positive and negative directions produced a positive, non-zero average. The results of these calculations were plotted on a graph of force versus angle of attack.

An interesting observation during the drag test was that once the angle of attack surpassed −20 degrees, the wake left by the tail of the ski also began to change noticeably. At −25 degrees a trail of white water emanated from the center of the ski tail. When the angle was increased to −30 degrees, water actually began to spout up from underneath the ski tail. As an angle increased again to −35 degrees, a rooster tail began to form from the ski tail, and fanned out as it passed behind the ski.

The outdoor test was designed to verify that the apparatus could collect data at higher speeds (at least 30 mph) and to generate a wing angle versus drag curve from a speeding boat. The equipment used for the outdoor drag test included a Connelly Performance Series FX ski, a ski clamp, 100 lbf load cell, ski boat, a strain indicator, an AD card, a TI laptop computer, an 8 ft plank with heavy eyelet, and nylon line.

The setup was essentially the same as the indoor test except that instead of having the transducer push the ski through the water (as from the two carriage), the force measured was the tension in the rope attaching the ski to the boat. Otherwise, the load cell was calibrated as before. Tests were to be taken from −5 degrees to −35 degrees.

The next phase in the verification was to waterproof the *MOSES* system components. The procedure was to simply strip *MOSES* down to just the waterproof compartments, immerse the system in water and bang it around, trying to dislodge the coverings. The system was then checked for moisture upon removal.

Once the system was proved safe for the electronics to be near water, the servo test could take place. The objective for the servo drag test was to generate drag curves, using first the tow tank and then the outdoor test, that could be compared to the fixed wing curves generated previously. The system setup was exactly the same as in the indoor and outdoor drag test, except that the *MOSES* system is activated and moves the wing from −5 degrees to −20 degrees during the run.

The last phase of the verification was to be the comprehensive test. Unfortunately, the test could not be run due to outdoor testing failures.

Evaluation

The *MOSES* system was fabricated and tested as an addition to standard slalom skis that will improve the drag characteristics of the ski, improving slalom performance. An analysis of the tests performed on *MOSES* starts in the following sequence: waterproofing, indoor testing, and outdoor testing.

The waterproofing of the *MOSES* system was quite successful as far as the core electronics were concerned. The use of modified Tupperare and rubber gaskets proved to be quite efficient in terms of sealing out water and in terms of getting extra performance per limited monetary resources. The inside came up bone dry after immersion.

The indoor testing of *MOSES* also proved pleasing to the team. The apparatus was able to take data from the ski with the wing fixed in position.

The indoor testing of the servo also worked out well. *MOSES* is able to push the wing around as the ski is traveling at 8.2 mph.

The outdoor drag test was just short of disaster. The good part of the test was that nothing broke (except one weak length of line). No electronics were shorted out, but the ski was highly unstable in that test setup. The amount of noise generated as the ski bounced around at the side of the boat made it impossible to collect useful data. Also, the ski was jolted so vigorously by the movements of the boat and by the waves that there was great danger of the ski striking the boat (which did not belong to either member of the *MOSES* team). The test was aborted.

Due to the failure of the outdoor apparatus to generate data in the fixed wing situation, the *MOSES* system was not strapped on to try to move the wing at 30 mph. There would be no experimental curve to compare to, so there was no point in risking the system to damage. No comprehensive test was performed for the same reasons. Putting a human test dummy on the *MOSES* system without knowing if it functioned would result in hurting the system or the person or both.

Conclusions and Recommendations

The indoor testing of the *MOSES* system found a system working flawlessly. Unfortunately, flawless performance at 8.2 mph does not really mean success in improving ski performance. Professional skiers have a velocity range of 20 to 70 mph, with the drag and lift forces on the wing at maximum velocity being quite intimidating from a design standpoint. Unless a true test could be performed at a minimum of 32 mph, the true extent of the *MOSES* system capabilities cannot be known.

Shortcomings in the design of the prototype include the waterproofing of the servo. The use of ziplock bags is not the greatest solution to protecting the most expensive electrical component (except in the sense of weight). The constant replacement of bags took much time during testings and many near heart-attacks were experienced by the designers every time the system became completely immersed (is it going to live through this?).

Another problem noticed late in the project was the change in balance of the ski. Adding the *MOSES* system, especially the battery, to the rear of the ski changed the balance characteristics of the ski, which would invariably change the "feel" of it when a skier was trying to take a turn. In a slalom course, if the ski is not balanced correctly so that the skier can lean forward or backward quickly, the skier is going to have no control of acceleration or deceleration and will most likely fall. The solution to this is simple; add weight to the tip of the ski until the balance character of the ski is restored to factory settings. The bindings can be moved for this purpose in conjunction with adding weight. Finding the correct balance point is impossible without skiing on the ski. Measurements only go so far, eventually, someone has to ski it to see if it's right or not.

The biggest setback as far as meeting the test objectives came in the failure of the outdoor drag test. We did not have an adequate setup for getting drag data at 30 mph, with or without the *MOSES* system installed. There was simply too much noise when dragging just a light waterski behind or to the side of a speedboat at those kinds of velocities. Since the test was performed late due to weather difficulties, team *MOSES* had very little time to recover from this testing failure. An alternative setup could not be manufactured in time, thus leaving no choice but to forego the comprehensive test as well. The dangers of riding on the ski without prior drag data taken from an unmanned setup were just too great. The lack of a comprehensive test left the team without the important "feel" variable which cannot be quantified, but is crucial in determining whether improvements in performance have been made.

An alternative setup was clearly needed for the outdoor drag test. Now that the course is completed, it is obvious that a design review of the test plan and verification system could have saved the *MOSES* team from outdoor failure. It would have been great to have feedback from other teams on our plan. Perhaps someone would have pointed out how the ski would really behave at high speeds. Regrets aside, an alternative test apparatus has been proposed for any future testing in the field of waterski drag character. It is a three ski setup, two being made quickly from wood or cut down from antique skis to serve as stabilizers for the ski under test. The tested ski would be pushed by a bracket and a force transducer, much as the indoor setup was performed, instead of tension in the rope connecting the boat and the apparatus. The apparatus would be tied to the boat, and the cable connecting the transducer to the data acquisition hardware would wrap around the tow rope. The two stabilizing skis would attach via a simple bracket system. The ski is now fixed laterally, is being pushed rather than pulled, and can take much more of a beating from the fluid without cause for worry as far as damage to the test equipment or the ski components.

Project Organization and Management

Project Organization

Team *MOSES* is composed of Steff Kelsey and Greg Wolff and is advised by Dr. Dave Watt. Kelsey is the team leader and was responsible for organizing meetings, networking in the academic and industrial community, as well as design, fabrication, and testing duties. Wolff had design, fabrication, and testing duties, as well as some fundraising responsibilities.

Facilities

The *MOSES* team based operations out of Kingsbury Hall, Room 101. It was there that *MOSES* was assembled and waterproofed, as well as serving as the site for many team meetings. The drafting work for the *MOSES* design was done in the Mechanical Engineering computer cluster, Kingsbury Hall Room M223. All machine work was done in Kingsbury Hall room 118 under the supervision of Bob Champlin.

The bulk of the *MOSES* testing was performed at the UNH Ocean engineering building. Specifically, the tow tank was utilized to obtain low speed (under 10 mph) drag data as well as low speed verification. The OE tow tank consists of a 120 feet long, 8 feet wide, and 12 feet deep pool with tracks running along the edges. A cart rides along the tracks which can tow just about anything for 90 feet. The data acquisition system has twenty-four channels available to input data from strain gages or LVDTs. The system is run through a unique wireless LAN network with a transmitting range of 2,500 feet, enabling data to be gathered from anywhere in the building.

The rest of *MOSES* testing was performed at Bow Lake, courtesy of the Paine family. Team *MOSES* was given access to a 17-foot speed boat outfitted with a wakeboard tower, a slalom pole, and a driver (many thanks to Jim Paine). Team *MOSES* was also equipped with a strain indicator, a laptop computer with an analog to digital converter installed, and oscilloscope type software to gather the data.

Schedule

The major milestones for the project *MOSES* are as follows:
- Project Selection: 9/11
- Project Summary: 9/25
- Project Proposal: 10/15
- Decision Matrices   10/21
- Preliminary Design Review   10/23
- Reliability Analysis   11/9

- Final Design Review   12/6
- Final Design Report   12/13
- Design Verification Plan   4/14
- Final Design and Test Report   5/9

21 Sentimentality and the Writings of the French Revolution

Erica Thoits

Winner of the English Department's 2005 Edmund Miller Essay Prize
for a sample English writing guide see chapter 29

In eighteenth-century Britain, sentimentality was not reserved for things such as a Jane Austen novel or Olaudah Equiano's *The Interesting Slave Narrative*, but was also inexorably caught up with the writings on both sides of the French Revolution. Sentimentality permeated all types of writings of the period, and is even found in the polemic essays of Edmund Burke, Thomas Paine, and Mary Wollstonecraft. While Burke chose to utilize sentimentality to further sympathy for the French Royal Family and everything it stood for, Wollstonecraft and Paine criticized Burke for that very use. It is possible that precisely because the eighteenth-century was so saturated with popular sentimental writing that these authors felt compelled to follow along with the increasingly sentimental trends of their time in order to reach and cater to a wider audience.

Reading an example of sentimental language from Jane Austen's *Sense and Sensibility* is the perfect way to understand what sentimentality really denotes. Here, Marianne displays her sentimentality as she dramatically describes Norland:

'And how does dear, dear Norland look?' cried Marianne. 'Dear, dear Norland,' said Elinor, 'probably looks much as it always does at this time of year. The woods and walks thickly covered with dead leaves.' 'Oh!' cried Marianne, 'with what transporting sensations have I formerly seen them fall! How have I delighted, as I walked, to see them driven in showers about me by the wind! What feelings have they, the season, the air altogether inspired! Now there is no one to regard them. They are seen only as a nuisance, swept hastily off, and driven as much as possible from the sight.' (Austen 83)

That Marianne completely over-dramatizes something as simple as leaves falling in the autumn is exactly what sentimental language is all about; it is the overstatement of emotions, pouring out one's heart at the slightest upset. Austen perfects the sentimental in the character of Marianne, and that sentimental writing is eventually borrowed by authors such as Burke, William Wilberforce, William Bodwin, and Olaudah Equiano.

As authors such as Burke, Paine, and Wollstonecraft demonstrate, sentimentality influenced politics of the day as well as fiction. Forms of sentimentality had an influence on the beginnings of the Revolution itself. Beth Lau writes in her introduction to Austen's novel *Sense and Sensibility* that:

Those who embraced Sensibility [. . .] believed that people are naturally good and benevolent [. . .] the emphasis on the goodness of all people and the celebration of nature over civilization would appear to have a democratizing effect, rendering people of all social ranks equal in their virtue and capacity for strong feeling. (Lau 3-4)

Lau goes on to say that these sentimental ideals are reminiscent of the work Jean Jacques Rousseau was doing in France. Ultimately, the thoughts of Rousseau would heavily influence the French Revolution, especially the belief that humanity is naturally good and only becomes corrupted by the falseness of social institutions. This idea is imbedded in the initial objectives of the Revolution that intended to deconstruct those very institutions and give the citizens of France "more freedom to act according to their natural desires" (Lau 3). Due to the fact that core principles of sentimentality are in agreement with Rousseau, many people at the time of the Revolution began to associate sentimentality with the massive upheaval occurring just across the channel in France (Lau 3-6).

Despite this relationship between revolution and sentimentality, Burke uses the language of authors such as Austen and Olaudah Equiano in his *Reflections on the Revolution in France* when describing the plight of Queen Marie Antoinette and her family as they are arrested by Parisian mobs:

From this sleep the queen was first startled by the sentinel at her door, who cried out to her, to save herself by flight— that this was the last proof of fidelity he could give—that they were upon him, and he was dead. Instantly he was cut down. A band of cruel ruffians and assassins, reeking with his blood, rushed into the chamber of the queen, and pierced with a hundred bayonets and poniards the bed, from whence this persecuted woman had but just time to fly almost naked, and through ways unknown to the murderers, had escaped to seek refuge at the feet of a king and husband, not secure of his own life at the moment. (Burke 809)

Burke goes on for a few more pages to describe the children of the Queen, her imprisonment, and the lack of chivalry surrounding her treatment at the hands of the unfeeling citizens. His detailed catalogue of events is comparable to Equiano's numerous descriptions of his maltreatment and despair that occur throughout the narrative. For instance, when Equiano is being deserted and betrayed by Captain Doran, Equiano writes: "I followed them with aching eyes as long as I could, and when they were out of sight I threw myself on the deck, with a heart ready to burst with sorrow and anguish" (Equiano 94). Burke heavily draws from the emotionally charged language that Equiano often uses.

Equiano's narrative is part of a group of writings that worked to further the Abolition cause in eighteenth-century Britain. William Wilberforce, when giving an anti-slavery speech, also employs sentimentality in the passage below in his *A Letter on the Abolition of the Slave Trade*:

Conceive, if you can, the agony with which, as he is hurried away by his unfeeling captors, he looks back upon the native village which contains his wife and children who are left behind, or, supposing them to have been carried off also, with which he sees their sufferings, and looks forward to the dreadful future, while his own anguish is augmented by witnessing theirs. (Wilberforce 72)

After reading Equiano's narrative and Wilberforce's *Letter*, both of which were written for political reasons, it is easy to see where Burke could have witnessed the use of sentimentality for political writings.

Even the anti-government and law novel *Caleb Williams* by William Godwin uses the language of sentimentality to further a political cause. The character of Emily Melville, a victim of tyranny and the abuse of law, is a perfect example of the sentimentality that Godwin employs. As she lies dying in a bed, a situation that is highly reminiscent of Marianne's illness in *Sense and Sensibility*, her nurse Mrs. Hammond is described here:

> She loved her like a mother. Upon the present occasion, every sound, every motion, made her tremble. Doctor Wilson had introduced another nurse in consideration of the incessant fatigue Mrs. Hammond had undergone, and he endeavored by representations and every authority to compel her to quit the apartment of the patient. But she was uncontrollable. (Goodwin 91)

This dramatic illness and Mrs. Hammond's refusal to leave Emily's bedside is a perfect example of how Godwin uses the sentimentality of the time to talk about such things as tyranny and the various abuses of the law. Godwin's novel, combined with the abolitionist writings alone, provide a large example of what Burke was doing: using the literary language of the day to write a political essay.

All of these political discourses utilize language that is seen in Austen's novels of the time. Since all of this sentimental language was being borrowed from the literature of the time for political writings, it is hardly surprising that Burke would join the trend he could not help but see forming around him. The use of sentiment is precisely what Paine and Wollstonecraft find so inappropriate.

Both authors severely criticize Burke for writing such a heightened emotional style. That they chose to attack Burke for his sentimental style is testament to how much attention sentimentality was receiving. In *The Rights of Man*, Paine's response to Burke's *Reflections*, Paine harshly writes of Burke's sentimental tendencies:

> As to the tragic paintings by which Mr. Burke has outraged his own imagination, and seeks to work upon that of his readers, they are very well calculated for theatrical representation, where facts are manufactured for the sake of show, and accommodated to produce, through weakness of sympathy, a weeping effect. But Mr. Burke should recollect that he is writing history, and not *plays*; and that his readers will expect truth, and not the spouting rant of high-toned exclamation. (Paine 849)

It is interesting that with all the political opinions Paine refutes, he chooses to take the time to include a section on Burke's use of the sentimental. According to Lau's introduction, many radicals such as Paine regarded sentimentality to be against the efforts of social reform because it "encouraged people to weep over suffering instead of actively working to alleviate it" (Lau 6). In Burke's view, the revolution was caused by irrational, brutal mobs, whereas Paine would see his radical cause as "characterized by its level-headed rationality and cool command of factual truth" (Lau 6). In a way, each author is accusing the other of being unreasonable and emotional. Burke is calling Paine and his revolutionaries crass and hotheaded, whereas Paine is leveling the same accusations right back at Burke.

Paine was not the only opponent of Burke's position on the Revolution and use of sentimentality in his *Reflections*; Mary Wollstonecraft also finds fault with Burke in *A Vindication of the Rights of Woman*. Wollstonecraft dislikes sentimentality for feminist reasons, shown here in a passage from her *Vindication*:

> Novels, music, poetry, and gallantry, all tend to make women the creatures of sensation, and their character is thus formed in the mould of folly during the time they are acquiring accomplishments [. . .] This overstretched sensibility naturally relaxes the other powers of the mind, and prevents intellect from attaining that sovereignty which it ought to attain to render a rational creature useful to others, and content with its own station [. . .] Another instance of that feminine weakness of character, often produced by a confined education, is a romantic twist of the mind, which has been very properly termed *sentimental*. (Wollstonecraft 318-320)

Sentimentality, for Wollstonecraft, is something that promotes weakness and intellectual inferiority in women. Wollstonecraft obviously held a negative preconceived notion of sentimentality; for Burke to use sentimentality in his attack on the supporters of the revolutionaries and the revolutionaries themselves would naturally automatically offend Wollstonecraft.

Wollstonecraft does not rely on a general refutation of sentimentalism, but here she directly attacks Burke's use of that mode of thought:

> But it is not very extraordinary that *you* should, for throughout your letter you frequently advert to a sentimental jargon, which has long been current in conversation, and even in books of morals, though it never received the *regal* stamp of reason. A kind of mysterious instinct is *supposed* to reside in the soul [. . .] This instinct, for I know not what other name to give it, has been termed *common sense*, and more frequently sensibility; and, by a kind of *indefeasible* right, it has been *supposed*, for rights of this kind are not easily proved, to reign paramount over the other faculties of the mind, and to be an authority from which there is no appeal. (Wollstonecraft 924)

Wollstonecraft, in the passages above, criticizes sentimentality as something that is insubstantial and imaginary; therefore, Burke cannot possibly base his anti-revolutionary arguments upon it. Burke is merely hiding behind his sentimental "jargon" because he lacks valid, tangible reasons for his assault on the French Revolution. Wollstonecraft even writes that Burke is "smearing a sentimental varnish over vice to hide its natural deformity" (Wollstonecraft 923). In Wollstonecraft's view, sensibility is a double evil: firstly because it promotes the inferiority of women, and secondly because Burke, in her opinion, uses it to disguise his weak argument when it comes to the Revolution.

Whether Burke was really hiding behind a veil of sentimentality, using it as a tool to gain the attention of an audience acclimated to sentimentality, or actually so truly horrified at the Queen's treatment that he could not filter out the emotion in his essay, both Paine and Wollstonecraft quite viciously attack him for his use of this style of writing. Undeniably much of the literature of the eighteenth-century, both political and fictional, employed the style of sentimentality one way or the other. It seems most likely that Burke was influenced by the writing of his time and chose to approach sections of his essay in the way he thought would be most widely accepted by readers.

Works Cited

Austen, Jane. *Sense and Sensibility*. Ed. Beth Lau. Boston: Houghton Mifflin Company, 2002.

Burke, Edmund. *Reflections of the Revolution in France*. 1790. *British Literature 1640-1789: An Anthology*. 2nd ed. Ed. Robert Demaria, Jr. Oxford: Blackwell Publishers, 2001. 803- 813.

Equiano, Olaudah. *The Interesting Slave Narratives and Other Writings*. Ed. Vincent Caretta. 4th ed. London: To. Wilkins, 1789; USA: W. Durell, 1791. New York: Penguin Books, 2003.

Lau, Beth. Introduction. *Sense and Sensibility*. By Jane Austen. Boston: Houghton Mifflin Company, 2002. 1-21.

Paine, Thomas. *The Rights of Man*. 1791. *British Literature 1640-1789: An Anthology*. 2nd ed. Ed. Robert Demaria, Jr. Oxford: Blackwell, 2001. 848-850.

Wilberforce, William. *A Letter on the Abolition of the Slave Trade*. 1870. *British Literature 1780-1830*. Ed. Anne K Mellor and Richard E. Matlak. Fort Worth: Harcourt Brace College Publishers, 1996. 71-73.

Wollstonecraft, Mary. *A Vindication of the Rights of Woman*. *British Literature 1640-1789: An Anthology*. 2nd ed. Ed. Robert Demaria, Jr. Oxford: Blackwell, 2001. 923-924.

22

Reformation Era Agitprop: Printed Propaganda, Class Consciousness and the Peasants' War

John C. Carroll

**Winner of the
History Department's 2005 Greenleaf Prize**

In 1523, shortly before the outbreak of the peasant revolts that would rock the southwestern portions of the Holy Roman Empire, a satirical dialogue was published which involved a wealthy *Bürger*, a priest and a farmer. Having been accused of usury by the peasant, the moneylender enlisted the aid of the priest in clearing his name, and the farmer countered their combined attack with a handful of passionate and incisive words: "Who gave you power? It seems you have a different God than we poor people."[1] This statement clearly shows that the issue at stake in this fictional argument was not merely the legality of lending money, which was the author's intended target, but the very right of certain classes to enjoy certain privileges and positions of power. From this exchange it is apparent that the lower classes of southwestern Germany and northern Switzerland were by this time quite aware of their social position within the feudal hierarchy, and the acrimonious tone of the retort suggests the violent conflict to come.

Suffering from a serious economic recession and smarting under the abuses of the clergy and nobility, the poor of the cities and both landed and landless peasants expressed their dissatisfaction and sought change for several years leading up to 1524. Appealing to local nobles against the clergy, regional courts against the nobles, and sometimes the Holy Roman Emperor himself, Southwestern Germany's underclass sought to reduce the power of the Catholic Church, punish or at least stop princely abuses

---

[1] Anonymous, *Zwiegespräch zwischen einem Bauern, einem reichen Bürger, einem Pfaffen und einemMönch über den Wucher*, in *Quellen zur Geschichte des deutschen Bauernstandes der Neuzeit*, ed., Franz Günter (Wissenschaftliche Buchgesellschaft, 1963, pg. 12.

and secure a free position for themselves.[2] Although some of these issues had been developing for over a half-century, Martin Luther's Reformation campaign infused these social reform movements with a strongly religious flavor.[3] This fusing of increasingly radical social aims with religious ideas that were nothing if not revolutionary completed the formula for one of the most interesting popular uprisings in European history. The general anti-clerical sentiments of peasants and artisans made them particularly susceptible to Reformation ideas, and once the institution of the Church was challenged using Biblical texts, the whole of society was subject to questioning. When the peasants of the Schwarzwald region revolted, compatriots in northern Switzerland, Saxony, Thuringen and Tyrol joined them within six months.[4] Although eventually defeated and subjected to a bloody repression, the rural and urban lower classes that participated in this uprising revealed a population able to inform, agitate and organize itself, independent of nobles, scholars or clergymen. Motivated by intense religious fervor and a strong sense of class solidarity that crossed the internal borders of the Holy Roman Empire, these craftsmen and farmers attempted to realize a new "community of Christ," based on Christian brotherhood and total equality. That this effort failed makes it no less fascinating or important to our understanding of Reformation-Era Germany.

The mass actions on the part of peasants and the urban underclass during the 1520s are evidence enough of increased social awareness and a rise in class consciousness: the publication of peasants' grievances, the fielding of armies made up almost entirely of farmers and poor artisans, the overthrow and murder of nobles and bishops are all indicative of a broad social movement. Printed propaganda played a pivotal role in fostering the development of this class-consciousness, which reached across the internal political and geographic boundaries of the Holy Roman Empire. Examination of the letters, accounts and pamphlets from the period reveals a society in turmoil and a militant movement for radical change. How much of a hand did the prodigious number of pamphlets, broadsides and flyers have in the development of a cohesive, regional class-consciousness among the lower castes? In what ways did these objects reflect the growing self-awareness of artisans and farmers? How far did these printed

---

[2] Paul A. Russell, *Lay Theology in the Reformation* (Cambridge: Cambridge University Press, 1986), pg. 114.

[3] James Stayer, *The German Peasants' War and Anabaptist Community of Goods*, (Montreal: McGill-Queen's University Press, 1991), pg. 35

[4] Stayer, pg. xi.

144 • Section 2

texts and images go in effecting a higher state of socio-economic awareness among "common man" readers?

In exploring this aspect of the German Reformation I will draw upon previous scholarly works on the use of flyers, illustrations and pamphlets in western and central Europe. However, this essay represents an effort to steer a middling course in contributing to a fuller understanding of the Peasants' War. I have heeded the advice of Geoffrey Dickens in the course of the research for, and writing of, this paper: "we . . . should not be overwhelmed by the presence of Martin Luther," nor should we simply parrot "the time-honoured Marxist obsession with the Peasants' Revolt."[5] It is important not to over-emphasize particularly productive pamphleteers, nor to politicize them by imposing present-day paradigms of social and political activity. Also, because these uprisings were so intricately intertwined with the religious movement of the day, the rise of a socially self-aware underclass in this period can only be fully understood by taking theological and religious issues into account. Although many works were principally concerned with the reform of the church, baptism or other religious debates, it is possible to tease out class attitudes and outlooks of both the writers and subjects in these pieces of popular writing. Moreover, this is a study of pamphlets and broadsides as objects, and an examination of their role as media for the dissemination of ideas and information among the lower classes. This is a relatively unexplored angle of sixteenth century popular social history in which the "Great Men" of the period will play only a small role: the focus is centered primarily on the writings by and/or for the poor urban artisans and rural farmers that made up the rank-and-file of this movement.

In examining the effects of such printed propaganda on popular consciousness it is necessary to analyze both the textual and visual contents of these works. The verbal imagery, word choice and proposals put forth in pamphlets would have elicited particular results given the medium through which they were presented and the content of the pamphlets merits close examination. Still, it must be recognized that it is quite easy to attribute far too much importance to the written arguments and assertions made in these booklets. In a society where at best only a tenth of the population was literate it is of key importance to emphasize the effects of the illustrations and symbols planted in pamphlets of the time. Before

---

[5] Geoffrey Dickens, "Intellectual and Social Forces in the German Reformation," in *Stadtbürgertum und Adel in der Reformation*, ed., Wolfgang Mommsen, Peter Alter and Robert Scribner (Stuttgart: Klett-Cotta, 1979), pgs. 11, 18.

moving on to these tasks, however, the role of pamphlets and broadsides should be defined, and the ways in which they were used examined.

In dealing with printed material from this time it is worthwhile to remember that such pieces of propaganda represented, in the words of historian Bernd Moeller, "a new, never-before-seen phenomena."[6] For the first time in history flyers, pamphlets and articles were mass-produced for a general audience, "the authors were contemporaries, the contents [of the works] of burning immediacy, their purpose to disseminate opinions [and] convictions."[7] The impact of these works on the consciousness and outlook of common laborers and farmers was far more pronounced than among the print-weary members of our society, regardless of whether the contents were read first hand or transmitted orally by an intermediary.

Despite the introduction of the printing press into German society, books remained costly and unattainable items for large segments of the population. Even after the pace of print production began to pick up, books remained objects of prestige among the lower ranks of society.[8] Still, texts were certainly available and the ubiquity and accessibility of written material in the early 1500s was truly extraordinary when compared to previous centuries. As Miriam Chrisman observed in her study of Sixteenth Century Stuttgart, *Lay Culture, Learned Culture*, almost half the population possessed books, including blacksmiths, fishermen and day laborers.[9] Given this information, it is safe to assume that many individuals among the lower classes would have been able to afford the considerably less expensive pamphlets, not to mention the broadsides, which one could peruse for free. Indeed, from the perspective of the writers and publishers who sought to stir up rebellious sentiment among the peasants and urban poor the pamphlet was the ideal medium. These could be produced in large numbers with great speed and sold for a fraction of the price of books. At the start of the century there were approximately forty editions of works in German published each year, but in 1523 the number of new volumes being produced had risen to 498.[10] We can infer from this that the aforementioned types of printed works would have enjoyed a

---

[6] Bernd Moeller, "Stadt und Buch," in *Stadtbürgertum und Adel in der Reformation*, pg. 30.

[7] Ibid., pg. 31.

[8] Chrisman, Miriam, *Lay Culture, Learned Culture: 1480-1599* (Yale University Press, 1982), pg. 71.

[9] Chrisman, pgs. 69-70.

[10] Scribner, Robert. *For the Sake of Simple Folk: Popular Propaganda for the German Reformation* (Cambridge: Cambridge University Press, 1981), pg. 2.

similar boom. Exemplary is the case of Strasbourg, where fifty-eight po-
lemics by laymen were published between 1520 and 1525.[11] An example
of the sheer quantity of items being produced comes to us from Leipzig
where one record showed that 1500 broadsheets attacking one Jerome
Emser were confiscated by authorities.[12]

Most pamphlets were short, encompassing little more than a dozen
pages, including the cover and title pages, which would have made them
far more accessible to the common reader. This brevity also helped contribute to the convenience and mobility of pamphlets, whose dimensions
were usually no more than 7 inches x 5 inches, roughly speaking, and took
up less than 42 square inches of surface space when laid flat.[13] Broadsides
tended to take up about three times this surface space, but they were only
one sheet thick, and could either be rolled or stacked flat. This made
transporting these items relatively easy: stacks of dozens or even hundreds
of pamphlets and broadsides could be distributed over several square miles
within a day, and much further within a week. The unassuming size of
pamphlets also made them easy to conceal and hide, when necessary.
When printers were closed down or forced underground, their pamphlets
survived them in many cases, and when city councils or nobles made efforts to confiscate or destroy radical popular literature, they rarely met
with much success. While Lutheran books burned, most pamphlets evad-
ed the fires.[14] Even in cities or rural areas where local authorities were on
the watch for such activity, such booklets would pass right under their
noses. Broadsides were more difficult to distribute, as they were usually
posted along major thoroughfares. This sort of activity was not forbidden
until after the Peasants' War, however, and during this period the fortunes
of many radical figures rose and fell based on such public propaganda.[15]
The sturdiness of the booklets certainly contributed to their success and is
attested to by their survival to the present. Although the examples available to present-day scholars certainly do not represent the majority of the
pamphlets printed, they are nevertheless impressive in their numbers.
While conscientious preservation on the part of various individuals de-

---

[11] Chrisman, pg. 157.

[12] Ibid., pg. 5.

[13] Observations based on two pamphlets by Thomas Mürner and Johnann
Eberlin von Günzberg, available at Harvard's Houghton Library.

[14] Günther Franz, *Der Deutsche Bauernkrieg* (Darmstadt: Hermann Gentner
Verlag, 1965), pg. 99.

[15] Scribner, "The Reformation as a Social Movement," in *Stadtbürgertum und
Adel in der Reformation*, pg. 57.

serves its due credit, the remarkable thickness and durability of the paper these publishers used guaranteed that the items would not wither to dust even long after the death of their creators.[16] This was certainly not an absolute necessity, as the subject matter of many of these pamphlets would have been outdated within years, if not months, but it made certain that this agitational literature reached its audience.

The question remains, however: how many people would have been able to read these pamphlets? In fact, although the average literacy rate for rural areas of the Holy Roman Empire was likely only five percent, in the larger urban centers it reached thirty percent or higher among the lower classes.[17] Indicative of the desirability of reading skills among the urban populace is a sign produced by Hans Holbein the younger in 1516 for reading and writing lessons. Under the text, which emphasizes the value of literacy for accounting one's debts, there is a picture of three men around a table, one holding a page half-filled with text, another a stylus and the third apparently instructing the two.[18] Not only were residents of southwestern German cities actively learning to read, the demand was so great that some literate individuals were able to make a profession out of relating this knowledge to others. Among the urban populace there was apparently both a will and a way to become part of the reading public.

The effect of the printed word was by no means lost on the dwellers of rural villages. Two major radical figures, Thomas Müntzer and Heinrich Pfeiffer, placed great importance on gaining the support of the village surrounding their Mühlhausen power base, and sent a series of articles to each village in the surrounding area. One could infer from the speediness with which they undertook this task that they had no doubt that the information would be distributed to the inhabitants and that at least some of them were literate.[19] Similarly, many of the dialogues published in the period preceding the Peasants' War involved farmers participating in quite literate discussions. Although rarely portrayed as being particularly bright, and representing just as much the Reformers' idealized vision of the peasant, the ubiquity of these characters seems to indicate that a good

---

[16] Observations of the above-mentioned pamphlets, available in the Houghton Library at Harvard.

[17] Chrisman, pg. 69.

[18] A painted sign advertising a schoolteacher's business, reprinted in *Lay theology in the Reformation*, Paul A.Russell, pg. 32.

[19] Tom Scott and Robert Scribner, *The German Peasants' War* (London: Humanities Press International, 1991), pg. 103.

number of peasants were able to read to some degree and that they were engaging others in discussion.[20]

Underlining the ways in which peasants actively engaged the information they received were the various communities that drew up articles, constitutions and ordinances. These Peasants' Assemblies and village councils also sent announcements, proposals and other messages to each other in the form of broadsides and pamphlets meant not only to inform, but also to move recipients to action. In May of 1525, for example, Black Forest Peasants proposed a boycott of Lords and clergy who resided in castles and monasteries, the aim being to force them from these highly defensible positions. One proposal was sent to Villingen to be posted around the town center and distributed among the populace. That the Peasants who composed this "call to action" expected some kind of active participation on the part of the recipients is reflective of exactly how powerful the printed word could be—the advocates of this boycott knew to whom they should address and send their ideas, and seem to have fully expected cooperation.[21]

This raises an important and obvious question, however: how did the radical message in these writings reach the illiterate? This was not an oversight by the authors or publishers; rather, it was an accepted social convention of the time that these pieces would be read aloud, often in public.[22] Lay preachers became a fixture of the rural and urban landscapes during this period, and it was common for these "street-preachers" to repeat sermons published by more prominent figures of the Reformation, Luther chief among them. The authors themselves were quite aware of the value of preaching, and for many printing seemed more a supplement to this task than an end in itself. In fact, aside from speaking at public gatherings or in village squares, these Reformation proselytizers often performed these sermons in Catholic Churches taken over by unruly townsfolk.[23] Here, perhaps playing on the traditionally revered and awe-inspiring setting, many diatribes against the clergy and the nobility were

---

[20] Anonymous, *Ein schöner Dialogus Cunz und Fritz*, in *Die Sturmtruppen der Reformation*, ed. Arnold F. Berger (Verlag von Phillip Reclam, 1931), pgs. 164-165.

[21] Stayer, pgs. 54-55.

[22] Steven Ozment, "Pamphlets as a Source. Comments on Bernd Moeller's 'Stadt und Buch,'" in *Stadtbürgertum und Adel in der Reformation*, pg. 46.

[23] Scribner, "The Reformation as a Social Movement," in *Stadtbürgertum und Adel in der Reformation*, pg. 57.

delivered, some of which incited vandalism or violence, as in Constance in June of 1524.[24]

Among the peasants there were also numerous ways in which the textual messages of these pamphlets and broadsides could be spread orally to others, sometimes under the cover of other activity. Johannes Kessler, who chronicled the development of the Twelve Articles years after the end of the uprising, described how disgruntled peasants roamed about the countryside to inform their compatriots under the pretense of exchanging *Fastnacht* holiday gifts:

> *". . . During Carnival time, when it is custom to assemble, six or seven met in Baltringen, a village near Ulm, and discussed many things about the difficult times. Then, as was the peasant custom at this time, they marched around from one village to another to their neighbors, in order to eat and drink in good company together, and the peasants of one village marched along with them to the next. If anyone asked what they were doing or what they wanted, they replied, 'We are fetching the carnival cakes from one another."*[25]

For the illiterate the visual components of pamphlets and broadsheets served to provide an idea of the text's subject matter and influence their opinion. The placement of images in pamphlets was virtually universal—not a single one examined in the research for this paper was without one. Broadsheets consisted primarily of pictorial items, since they needed to catch the eyes of passersby in order to attract their attention to the finer details of the illustrations and the text which accompanied them. The broadsides were thus used much like the placards and posters of today: they were consciously placed in, over, opposite or next to places where eyes would be likely to land on them. In this way such propaganda actually became a part of the landscape, lining the thoroughfares and adorning the public and private structures, perhaps affecting the populace on even a subliminal level as they became accustomed to these images and symbols.

Now that the role and uses of pamphlets and broadsides has been examined, let us consider what was transmitted through such media. The fact that such literature was available to the urban and rural underclass

---

[24] Veit Suter, *Letter to Archduke Ferdinand from the Austrian Roving Ambassador*, in *The German Peasants' War*, ed. Tom Scott and Robert Scribner, pg. 122.

[25] Johannes Kessler, *Sabbata*, in *The German Peasants' War*, ed. Tom Scott and Robert Scribner, pg. 122.

does not in and of itself shed light on the development of their collective class awareness; rather, it merely opens up the possibility that printed propaganda played a role in developing and sustaining class-consciousness among the populace. We must now examine the content of these works in order to determine how such printed material would have influenced the attitudes and outlook of peasants and artisans during this period.

Peasants were attracted to the Reformation and to the figure of Martin Luther from a very early stage. As a character in one dialogue from 1521 put it, "he who possesses many benefices is the enemy of Luther . . . but the poor masses love him dearly."[26] During these last years before the revolts broke out the content of most pamphlets were not particularly radical, but a special focus of all Reformation pamphleteers was on the 'common' people. In fact, it is a good indication of the effects of this popular literature that many among the lower ranks of German society became authors themselves, encouraged by the likes of Huldrych Zwingli.[27] In his examination of eight pamphlet writers from Southwestern Germany, Paul A. Russell analyzed the written works of weavers, housewives, furriers, painters and shoemakers.[28] One, Sebastian Lotzer, was a fairly prominent pamphleteer in Memmingen who published a half dozen booklets between 1523 and 1525.[29] Although he often worded his pieces carefully, so as not to appear to be inciting rebellion, this furrier's works were filled with condemnation for "disgusting papists" who persecuted evangelical preachers and denunciations of those who oppressed the poor, be they religious or secular authorities.[30] Another, Utz Rychssner, a weaver from Augsburg, wrote a dialogue involving two members of his own class, one a weaver who convinces the other character to turn his back on the church. Rychssner also defended the rights of the poor, in particular the right to preach.[31] The case of these urban craftsmen illustrate a number of important points: one, that the writings of Reformation leaders and scholars, whether of a more moderate or radical leaning, had found purchase in the fertile soil of the urban lower class; two, that a concept of a common identity among artisans and peasants, the latter of whom were often defended in these pamphleteers' writings, had begun to develop;

---

[26] Anonymous, *Ein schöner Dialogus Cunz und Fritz*, in *Sturmtruppen der Reformation*, pg. 165.

[27] Paul A. Russell, pg. 68.

[28] Ibid., pg. 10.

[29] Ibid., pg. 90.

[30] Ibid., pg. 94, 96.

[31] Ibid., pg. 125.

and finally, that these artisans began to "produce for their own," that is to say, they were now writing with farmers and craftsmen in mind. Despite the milder tone of some of these works, the very fact that members *of* the lower class were writing *for* the lower class points to the development of a strong socio-economic identity.

By the time these pamphlets were published, however, increasingly extreme ideas and proposals were appearing with regularity. Two pieces by Johann Eberlin von Günzberg published in 1521 are representative of both the 'mainstream' and radical sides of the Reformation. In his *Pitiable Petition to the Holy Roman Emperor*, von Günzberg presents the grievances of the common people to the Emperor, claiming that they have no one else to turn to.[32] Appealing to the Emperor's own desire for greater independence from Rome, von Günzberg derides the "barefoot, begging mendicant monks" as parasites, and claims that the Vatican and the monastic orders deploy hundreds of thousands of Guldin every year as part of their efforts to maintain control of the Holy Roman Empire.[33] He goes on to blame the church for the shortage of specie in Germany during this period, claiming "Rome sucks up all silver and gold."[34] Aside from addressing his concerns to the Imperial Crown, this petition by von Günzberg is fairly tame in other ways as well. It appeals to the nascent German nationalism that grew during this period, defending Luther and Ulrich von Hutten as "German-born, learned and Christian men."[35] Likewise, the attacks on the Church were by this time old news; despite the high level of popular anticlericalism, this piece fails to address directly any of the issues connected to the Church's role in the lives of the peasants or city-dwellers; instead it limits itself entirely to issues that would have resonated with a more privileged audience.

If his 'open-letter' to the Emperor represented a calculatingly moderate petition to a royal authority, von Günzberg's dialogue from the same year, *It is a wonder to me that there is no money in the land*, was an unapologetic indictment of the groups that were considered antagonistic to the "common man." In this piece a handful of characters assign the blame for the economic difficulties of period to a host of enemies. One participant in the dialogue attributes the hardships of the people to the lords and lesser nobles, who allow their servants to carry out campaigns of rape and

---

[32] Johann Eberlin von Günzberg, *Ein klägliche Klag an die christliche Römischen Kaiser Carolum...*, (Basel:Pamphilus Gegenbach, 1521), pgs. 1-2.

[33] Ibid., pgs. 4-6.

[34] Ibid., pg. 9.

[35] Ibid., pg. 3.

pillage while they turn a blind eye. Their taste for opulence and finery are also named as cause for the impoverishment of the commoners, and he charges that nobles import "plenty of pretty clothes and good Crowns from France."[36] Another character in the dialogue blames merchants and competition from foreign craftsmen: "See, in our German land we have enough people to fill all the necessary crafts, we have all the necessary materials . . . iron, gold silver . . . wine, corn . . . cattle, birds, fish, [etc.]. [But] we allow too many costly innumerable scarves, precious stones . . . wine and craftsmen to be brought to us from the Ends of the Earth."[37] Here, Eberlin von Günzberg has exchanged the role of mediator between the general populace and the crown for that of the champion of the commoners. Although no specific proposals or courses of action are put forward, the very assignment of guilt to the upper classes and clergy is itself radical, and the focus on economic factors reinforces the sense of social antagonism developed in the pamphlet.

This more socially extreme, class-based form of Reformation was also publicly advocated in a series of statements published by Eberlin von Günzberg's *Bund*, a group of over a dozen radicals that supported the Reformation and the Peasants' War in turn. Although some concern themselves primarily with the translation of the Bible into German or other fairly common Reformation-era issues, other members' statements were very forward thinking for the time.[38] The eleventh Member of the *Bund*, for example, proposes in his article that the sale of certain products be restricted in order to protect local craftsmen and farmers:

> "No wine that has not been produced in our land should be brought in.

> "No scarf that has not been made in our land should be brought in.

> "No fruit that did not grow in our land should be brought in."[39]

---

[36] Johann Eberlin von Günzberg, *Mich wundert das kein gelt [im] land ist* (Elyemburg: Jacob Stöckel, 1521), pg. 3.

[37] Ibid., pg. 251.

[38] Eberlin von Günzberg et al., *Artikeln der Bundisgenossen*, in *Die Sturmtruppen der Reformation*, pg. 135.

[39] Ibid., pg. 154.

This member also advises the urban populace to ensure that Master Craftsmen do not outnumber apprentices, so that "bad" competition does not impoverish the community.[40] These were issues firmly rooted among the lower classes, especially the artisans of the towns and city. These were subjects that would have resonated with individuals from these castes, and by addressing artisans and farmers as a common class, these statements had the potential to produce or reinforce a sense of collective identity, even one that covered both the rural and urban underclass.

Of equal, if not greater, importance to our understanding of the effects of these works are the illustrations that adorned them. The visual contents of broadsides and pamphlets would have carried considerable weight in a time and place where much of the target audience was illiterate. Still, while images and symbols are powerful and can be rendered in a very detailed manner, they are open to interpretation. The images used in the printed propaganda of this time were not mere decorations or additions to the text—they were central to the purpose of transmitting specific messages and ideas. While the printed word alone could potentially make clear the intentions of the author, this would have proven a vain exercise without pictorial accompaniment. For most peasants and artisans of the day, these illustrations would have been more meaningful and moving than the most subtle of points and passionate of passages. The publishers, authors and artists involved in the production of these pieces were certainly aware of the need to communicate their message through visual as well as textual media, and as a consequence these pictures often contain specific symbols, objects or themes which can be identified and decoded. This process allows us in turn to reconstruct the referential framework of peasants and artisans who interpreted these images.

A basic necessity for such visual propaganda would have been cues that allowed viewers to distinguish which groups or factions the individuals portrayed would have belonged to. In depicting members of the clergy or ecclesiastical and theological scholars a variety of related items and articles were used, any of which fulfilled the task of informing the audience about what side the individuals depicted stood on. On the cover of a dialogue published in 1524 in Speyer by one Jakob Fabri stand the four figures involved in the discussion related in the pamphlet: a farmer, the devil, Erasmus von Rotterdam and Johann Fabri. Here Erasmus von Rotterdam is shown jealously clutching an ornate papal crown, holding it close to his body with one arm and caressing it with his free hand.[41] An essentially identical crown was often shown in other illustrations in connection with

---

[40] Ibid., pg. 155.

various types of Church figures, bishops and the Pope chief among them. The cover illustration of Eberlin von Günzberg's aforementioned "open letter" to the Holy Roman Emperor also displayed the clergy in such a manner. Here the Pope is shown making an agreement with the devil, adorned with gold jewelry and accompanied by a retinue of similarly-clad bishops, one of whom is carrying an elaborate head-ornament bearing a strong resemblance to that appearing on the cover of the dialogue published by Jakob Fabri.[42] Likewise, antagonistic scholars, are often shown wearing clothes suggesting comfortable circumstances and with the implements of their profession. One illustration showing clergymen and a canon lawyer dressed in garments typical of their station under attack by peasants.[43] These figures were also frequently the subjects of satirical renditions: on the cover of the aforementioned dialogue Johann Fabri is depicted in expensive clothing with a parchment in one hand and a billow in the other—perhaps marking him as a blower of hot air.[44]

In a similar vein, urban patricians were usually wearing fine clothing in the woodcuts of the time, as in the image that appeared on a broadside by Hans Sachs in 1524. Here the furs and fine clothes of the wealthy burghers are contrasted directly with the simple, worn garb of two artisans, whose haggard faces compare poorly to the plump and condescending visages of their superiors.[45] The arrangement of the figures is such that the burghers even seem to be accosting their impoverished counterparts, and their antagonistic stances underline the picture's overall sense of tension. Likewise, Peter Fletner's *The Poor Common Ass* represents the common castes as a steed ridden hard by two human figures, tyranny and usury. The first character is a scepter-holding, armored noble, while the second presents a winged, well-dressed nightmarish banker.[46]

---

[41] Erasmus Alberus (?), Title page to *Gesprech büchlein von einem Bawern, Belial, Erasmo Rotteroda und doctor Johann Fabri*, reprinted in *Die Reformation im zeitgenössischen Dialog*, ed. Werner Lenk (Berlin: AkademieVerlag, 1968), pg. 243.

[42] Johann Eberlin von Günzberg, title page to *Ein klägliche Klag an die christliche Römischen Kaiser . . .* (Basel:Pamphilus Gegenbach, 1521), available from Houghton Library Collection, Harvard University.

[43] Woodcut from Joseph Grünpeck's *Spiegel*, reprinted in Paul A. Russell's *Lay Theology in the Reformation*, pg. 134.

[44] Erasmus Alberus(?), Title page, reprinted in *Die Reformation im zeitgenössischen Dialog*, pg. 243.

[45] Image from a broadside by Hans Sachs, in Paul A. Russell, *Lay theology in the Reformation*, pg. 34.

The inverse of these negative portrayals of the clergy and upper classes were the images that promoted farmers and artisans as protagonists in a just and pious struggle. The title page of a dialogue published in 1523-24 contained four figures, a monk, a priest, a "handworker" and a farmer. Here again we see contrasts in clothing and poise. The monk and the priest are both seated, before them lies an open backgammon board. The priest is well-dressed, but not to an overly extravagant degree, while the monk wears a simple habit. By contrast, the artisan wears a workman's cap and simpler clothing, while the peasant's garb is simplest of all, a small purse and a walking stick being his only adornments. In terms of physical attitude and positioning, the two clergymen are seated at an elevated table, which is positioned higher than the one the artisan is seated at. The peasant, who appears to be just entering, is the only one standing. While the clothing and seated station of the monk and priest seems to accent their social standing, it is interesting that the farmer is portrayed in such an active stance, standing tall and moving towards the group, perhaps indicative of the special spiritual strength accorded the peasantry by many Reformation writers.[47] More explicit examples of the "holy peasant" abound, however. The title woodcut from Diepold Peringer's *Ein Sermon von der Abgotterey* shows a peasant preacher with a rosary-like object in his right hand and his left assuming a didactic position.[48] Another title page from 1523 shows a peasant kneeling and praying, again underlining the famed piety of rural farmers.[49] These types of images were very important to the Peasants' War and the Protestant cause as a whole, as they lent credibility and justification to commoners' movement for social and religious transformation. The images of greedy, exploitative bishops, nobles and burghers served the important propagandistic purpose of vilifying the opponents of the movement, while portrayals of godly peasants and wronged artisans emphasized the righteousness of revolt.

Leading up to the uprisings of 1524-1525 the anger became almost palpable in many images, as increasingly violent images were deployed as part of the propaganda campaign that preceded the Peasants' War. A prominent figure in many of these illustrations is a highly symbolic figure from the *Bundschuh* Rebellions that took place at the turn of the century,

---

[46] Reprinted in Robert Scribner's *For the Sake of Simple Folk*, pg. 93.

[47] Title page from *Von der Wallfahrt im Grimmetal*, reprinted in *Die Reformation im zeitgenössischen Dialog*, pg. 241.

[48] Reprinted as the frontispiece to Paul A. Russell's *Lay Theology in the Reformation*.

[49] Title page from *Meditations on the Our Father*, reprinted in Russell, pg. 53.

"Karsthans." Portrayed alternately with a hoe (*Karst*), a threshing flail or a scythe, this character personified the rebellious spirit of both artisans and peasants, who identified with him as an expression of the resilience and courage of the "common man."[50] One woodcut shows Karsthans thrashing the clergy with a flail, another shows him attacking a knight while a peasant strikes down the pope with a sword.[51] Once the revolt was in full swing, the scenes produced on broadsides and pamphlets reached a pinnacle of violence and bloodiness. One image produced by Lucas Cranach in 1526 is typical: women and children are shown abusing, robbing and beating priests to death with farm tools, pikes and stones.[52] Another, which served as the cover to an address to the Peasants' Assembly, shows "Christian Farmers" opposite the "Romanist and Sophist" knights, cardinals and bishops while the pope hangs on a wheel set to skewer him upon the pikes of the peasants.[53] Thus, beginning in the early 1520s, violent illustrations became frequent accompaniments to broadsheets and pamphlets, making the idea of armed rebellion seem increasingly possible and foreshadowing the revolts of 1524-1525. When these finally broke out these pictures would have served to glorify the conduct of the insurgents as justified and righteous, while reinforcing the rebels' thirst for vengeance. In fact, the early portrayals of violent insurrection may have proven to be self-fulfilling prophesies, pictures that progressively accustomed readers and viewers to the idea of overthrowing the existing social system by force until it seemed like the obvious course, an inevitability.

There were also pictures envisioning a bright future for the craftsmen and farmers who took part in these uprisings. One piece shows the social order "turned on its head," as a priest and a bishop till the fields while a peasant celebrates mass within a church. In the lower left-hand corner of the picture a friendly artisan greets a man who appears ready to barter.[54] The title woodcut for *A Mirror for the Blind*, a pamphlet by an imperial soldier named Haug Marschalck, shows a blindfolded clergy unable to see a beaming vision of Christ that blesses a "common man" figure for his piety.[55] These were among a small but interesting group of illustrations that

---

[50] Russell, pgs. 48-49.

[51] Reprinted in Russell, pg. 49; Erhard Schoen, *Illustration for a Prognostic*, reprinted in Scribner, *For the Sake of Simple Folk*, pg. 126.

[52] Reprinted in Russell, pg. 186.

[53] Titelpage to *An die versamlung gemeyner Bawerschaft*, reprinted in Scribner, *For the sake of simple folk*, pg. 121.

[54] Woodcut from Joseph Grünspeck's *Spiegel*, reprinted in Russell, pg. 139.

[55] Titlepage to *A Mirror for the Blind*, reprinted in Russell, pg. 131.

sought to provide a visual representation of the future world proposed by the principal figures of the radical Reformation, promising a bright tomorrow to the commoners engaged in a difficult, bloody and ultimately vain struggle.

Both the textual and visual contents of these pamphlets and broadsides fostered the development of a regional, common class consciousness among the rural and urban underclass in a variety of ways. By addressing their writings to both peasants and artisans, pamphleteers of all stations helped produce a sense of common identity between these two groups, which had traditionally been considered distinct, mutually exclusive social units. The discussion of economic issues of direct concern to agriculture and to craftsmen reinforced a sense of social difference from the clergy, nobles and wealthy burghers, which were sometimes characterized as non-productive or parasitic classes in contrast to hard-working peasants and artisans. The vilification of aristocrats and bishops played upon existing antagonisms and would have only intensified the anger of the lower classes towards their superiors. In both the text and the illustrations of these pieces the social differences that existed in this part of the Holy Roman Empire are emphasized: positive virtues like piety and Christian fraternity are assigned to the lower classes while varied and sundry sinful acts become associated with the clergy, noblemen and urban patricians that held power. In more mundane ways pamphleteers promoted a sense of solidarity between the urban and rural lower classes, often tying their respective complaints and causes together by addressing them within the same booklet or poster and proposing similar solutions, as in the recommendations regarding trade and production by one of von Günzberg's *Bund*-members.

Delivered in a format that was capable of reaching a large audience, whether through direct distribution, lending and borrowing, or readings in public and private, these images and words were brought into direct contact with the segments of society targeted by the authors and publishers. When confrontation with the ruling segments of society became inevitable, it could be claimed that these works of printed propaganda were largely responsible for exacerbating the extant social tensions. Broadsides sent to villages and hinterlands exhorted community members to make common cause with their rebellious neighbors, while pamphlet illustrations glorified the armed struggle of peasants and presented images of a future utopian "Community of Christ" in which craftsmen and farmers would live together in pious harmony.

The power of these images and writings were magnified by the novel nature of such materials. Never before had so much material been printed and distributed among the general population. The subjects covered in these pieces were not being discussed "over the heads" of the lower castes, but were issues directly concerning and addressed to them. In fact, many authors' origins lay among the peasants and city-workers, a fact whose significance was certainly not lost on the target audience of these works. Indeed, the ability to lay hands on pamphlets that dealt with the "big issues" of the day was itself remarkable, and the reading public of this period would have been susceptible to such propaganda to a relatively high degree. The high rate of consumption was probably in part due to the agitation produced by such exciting events, but also likely a result of the novelty and relative newness of the popular press.[56] When the highly mobile and accessible pamphlets and broadsides were infused with radical content it had a marked effect; likewise, when issues pertaining to the situation of the urban and rural lower classes were presented through this medium, they were discussed across the region and gave impetus to the development of a common cause. Images portraying peasants and artisans as heroes or victims would have encouraged the audience to identify with the figures, and in turn, with each other as members of the same socioeconomic group. In any discussion pertaining to the development of class-consciousness in this region and period, the role of printed propaganda cannot be exaggerated.

While scholarly works considerable in number and scale have already dealt with this subject in detail, there remains plenty of latitude for academics seeking to refine our understanding of this turbulent and unique period in German history. In the realm of material culture there is still plenty of work to be done, especially with regards to the role of pamphlets. Moreover, new artifacts and information continue to be uncovered, promising new insight and perspective on the events of the period and the everyday lives of the people who experienced them. Drawing on the already prodigious body of historical literature on this period, future researchers will have a solid foundation on which to build their work, and I, for one, am interested to see what they produce.

Works Cited

Primary Sources
Alberus, Erasmus. *Gesprech büchlein von einem Bawern Belial, Erasmo Rotterodam vnd Doctor Johann Fabri, kürtzlich die warheyt anzeygend,*

---

[56] Robert Scribner, *For the Sake of Simple Folk: Popular Propaganda for the German Reformation*, pg. 2.

was Eraßmum vnd Fabrum zu verleugnung des gots worts bewegt hatt. In *Die Reformation im zeitgenössischen Dialog,* ed. Lenk, Werner, 215-223. Berlin: Akademie-Verlag, 1968.

Anonymous. *Ain grosser Preisz, so der Fürst der Hellen genant Lucifer den Gaystlichen Als Bäpst, Bischoff, Cardinel vnd der gleychen zuo weysst vnd empeüt . . .* Augsburg: M. Ramminger, 1521.

Anonymous. *Ein schöner Dialogus Cunz und Fritz.* In *Sturmtruppen der Reformation,* ed. Berger, Arnold F., 161-172. Leipzig: Verlag von Philipp Reclam, 1931.

Anonymous. *Ein Dialogus ader gesprech zwischen einem Vatter vnnd Sun, dye Lere Martini Luthers vnd sunst andere sachen des Cristlichen glaubens belangende.* In *Die Reformation im zeitgenössischen Dialog,* ed. Lenk, Werner, 151-167. Berlin: Akademie-Verlag, 1968.

Anonymous. *Die grundlichen und recten Hauptartikel aller Baurschaft und Hindersessen der gaistlichen und weltlichen Oberkaiten, von wölchen si sich beschwert vermeinen.* In *Quellen zur Geschichte des Bauernstandes,* ed. Franz, Günther, 14-19. Darmstadt: Wissenschaftliche Buchgesellschaft, 1963.

Eberlin von Günzberg, Johann, Members of the *Bundnisgenossen* (Anonymous). *Artikeln der Bundnisgenossen.* In *Sturmtruppen der Reformation,* ed. Berger, Arnold F., 125-160. Leipzig: Verlag von Philipp Reclam, 1931.

Eberlin von Günzberg, Johann. *Ein klägliche Klag an die christliche Römischen Kaiser Carolum wo wegte Doctor Luthers und Ulrich von Hutten . . .* Basel: Pamphilus Gegenbach, 1521. Available from the Houghton Collection, Harvard University.

_____. *Mich wundert das kein Geld [im] land ist.* Elyemburg: Jacob Stöckel, 1521. Available from the Baker Business Library, Harvard University.

Kessler, Johannes. *Sabbata* (Excerpt). In *The German Peasants' War,* ed. Scott, Tom and Scribner, Bob, 122-126. London: Humanities Press International, 1991.

Murner, Thomas. *Die disputacion vor den xij orten einer lobliche eidtgnoschafft nälich Bern . . .* Luzern: Publisher Unknown, 1527.

Suter, Veit. *Letter to Archduke Ferdinand.* In *The German Peasants' War,* ed. Scott, Tom and Scribner, Bob, 121-122. London: Humanities Press International, 1991.

Illustrations Cited

Cranach, Lucas. *Women Attack the Clergy.* In *Lay Theology in the Reformation*, Russell, Paul A., 186. Cambridge: Cambridge University Press, 1986.

Fletner, Peter. *The Poor Common Ass.* In *For the Sake of Simple folk*, Scribner, Robert, pg. 93. Cambridge: Cambridge University Press, 1981.

Woodcuts from Joseph Grünpeck's *Spiegel.* Reprinted in *Lay Theology in the Reformation*, Russell, Paul A., pgs. 134, 139. Cambridge: Cambridge University Press, 1986.

Title page to Haug Marschalck's *A Mirror for the Blind.* Reprinted in *Lay Theology in the Reformation*, Russell, Paul A., pg. 131. Cambridge: Cambridge University Press 1986.

Title woodcut from Diepold Peringer's *Ein Sermon von der Abgotterey.* Reprinted as the frontispiece to *Lay Theology in the Reformation*, Russell, Paul A. Cambridge: Cambridge University Press, 1986.

Image from a broadside by Hans Sachs. In *Lay Theology in the Reformation*, Russell, Paul A., pg. 34. Cambridge: Cambridge University Press, 1986.

Schoen, Erhard. *Illustration for a Prognostic* Reprinted in *For the Sake of Simple Folk*, Scribner, Robert, pg. 126. Cambridge: Cambridge University Press, 1981.

Title page to *An die versamlung gemeyner Bawerschaft.* Reprinted in *For the Sake of Simple Folk*, Scribner, Robert, pg. 121. Cambridge: Cambridge University Press, 1981.

Title page to *Ein klägliche Klag an die christliche Römischen Kaiser Carolum wo wegte Doctor Luthers und Ulrich von Hutten.* Basel: Pamphilus Gegenbach, 1521.

Title page to *Gesprech büchlein von einem Bawern, Belial, Erasmo Rotteroda und doctor Johann Fabri.* Reprinted in *Die Reformation im zeitgenössischen Dialog*, ed. Lenk, Werner, pg. 243. Berlin: AkademieVerlag, 1968.

Title page from *Von der Wallfahrt im Grimmetal.* Reprinted in *Die Reformation im zeitgenössischen Dialog*, ed. Lenk, Werner, pg. 241. Berlin: Akademie-Verlag, 1968.

Title page from *Meditations on the Our Father.* Reprinted in *Lay Theology in the Reformation*, Russell, Paul A., pg. 53. Cambridge: Cambridge University Press, 1986.

Secondary Sources

Chrisman, Miriam Usher. *Lay Culture, Learned Culture: Books and Social Change in Strasbourg, 1480-1599*. London and New Haven: Yale University Press, 1982.

Franz, Günther. *Der deutsche Bauernkrieg*. Darmstadt: Wissenschaftliche Buchgesellschaft, 1965.

_____. *Quellen zur Geschichte des Bauernstandes in der Neuzeit*. Darmstadt: Wissenschaftliche Buchgesellschaft, 1963.

Lenk, Werner. *Die Reformation im zeitgenössischen Dialog*. Berlin: Akademie-Verlag, 1968.

Mommsen, Wolfgang, P. Alter and R. Scribner. *Stadtbürgertum und Adel in der Reformation*. Stuttgart: Klett-Cotta, 1979.

Russell, Paul A. *Lay Theology in the Reformation: Popular Pamphleteers in Southwest Germany, 1521-1525*. Cambridge: Cambridge University Press, 1986.

Scott, Tom and Robert Scribner. *The German Peasants' War*. London and New Jersey: Humanities Press International, 1991.

Scribner, Robert. *For the Sake of Simple Folk*. Cambridge: Cambridge University Press, 1981.

Stayer, James M. *The German Peasants' War and Anabaptist Community of Goods*. Montreal: McGill-Queen's University Press, 1991.

Articles

Dickens, Geoffrey. "Intellectual and Social Forces in the German Reformation." In *Stadtbürgertum und Adel in der Reformation*, ed. Mommsen, W., P. Alter and R. Scribner. Stuttgart: Klett-Cotta, 1979.

Moeller, Bernd. "Stadt und Buch: Bemerkungen zur Struktur der reformatorischen Bewegung in Deutschland." In *Stadtbürgertum und Adel in der Reformation*, ed. Mommsen, W., P. Alter and R. Scribner. Stuttgart: Klett-Cotta, 1979.

Ozment, Steven. "Pamphlets as a Source: Comments on Bernd Moeller's 'Stadt und Buch.'" In *Stadtbürgertum und Adel in der Reformation*, ed. Mommsen, W., P. Alter and R. Scribner. Stuttgart: Klett-Cotta, 1979.

Scribner, Robert W. "The Reformation as a Social Movement." In *Stadtbürgertum und Adel in der Reformation*, ed. Mommsen, W., P. Alter and R. Scribner. Stuttgart: Klett-Cotta, 1979.

Section 3

Writing Assignments
from across the Disciplines

23

Writing Assignment

Dr. Rob Robertson

Introduction to Tourism (Tourism 400)

Assessment
of an Isle of Shoals Steamship Co. "Cruise" Experience

This assignment requires students to investigate, experience and formally evaluate a cruise aboard the Isles of Shoals Steamship Company's M/V Thomas Laighton. The goal of this assignment is to provide students the opportunity to critically assess a "tourism" experience. Students will investigate the various cruise options, select a cruise, take the cruise, and evaluate the overall "tourism" experience. Students will receive a complimentary cruise on any scheduled trip, including **Fall Foliage Tours of Great Bay and area rivers, Historic Isles of Shoals and Portsmouth Harbor Tours, Lighthouse Tours, Star Island Walkabout,** and **Party Ships** (21+ only). The complimentary cruise passport *does not include food and beverage or parking.* Guests of students will receive 50% off each ticket purchased by persons accompanying the student enrolled in the course (e.g., parents, friends, relatives).

This assignment requires a 6- to 8-page double-spaced (12-point font), 1 inch margins (this is the standard for all written assignments). In order to attain a satisfactory grade on this assignment it is expected that the paper include an introduction that allows the reader to understand the objectives of your paper and a conclusion that effectively summarizes the knowledge attained through the completion of this assignment. *This assignment is due approximately two weeks after your cruise experience.*

The Process

The following represents a description of the ticketing process. All students participating in this assignment must:

- Sign up for this assignment and receive a passport form from the teaching assistant.
- Make a reservation with the Isles of Shoal Steamship Company for the cruise experience that you will evaluate. Reservations may be made by phone or Internet.
- Turn in the completed passport/ticket for a boarding pass thirty minutes prior to departure.

The Assessment

This assessment of a tourist attraction requires the systematic collection of information about the entire experience from beginning to end. Your assessment must include the following components: (1) information search, (2) evaluation of alternatives and cruise selection, and (3) purchase and post-purchase evaluation. Your paper should address each of the following dimensions of each component:

Information Search. The goal of the section is to collect information and report information on three different cruise options offered by the ISSCO. Your written component provides a concise summary of what you think about each of the options. Your report should identify the source and describe the information obtained. You should use the following sources of information to complete your review and make your decision.

- *Personal Experience* (e.g., What does your personal experience tell you about each cruise option? Have you had prior experiences with ISSCO or a similar experience and recollections from other water-based excursion experiences?)
- *Isles of Shoals Steamship Brochure* (e.g., What did you learn about each of the cruises form the brochure? Was the brochure visually stimulating? How did the images make you feel? How would you rate the quality and quantity of information in the brochure? What information was missing? Did it provide enough information about each component?)
- *Isles of Shoals Steamship Company Web Site* (e.g., How easy was it to find the web site? How easy was it to navigate the web site? What was most useful in learning about the cruise options? How would you rate the quality and quantity of information on the web site? What information was missing?)

- *Personal Interviews with Four Different Target Audiences* (e.g., college students, parents, friends, co-workers). This source of information will help you learn about what other people think about each of the three cruise experience/options that you considered. Their opinions/comments can be based on prior experience, word of mouth, and/or personal opinions.

Evaluation of Alternative and Cruise Selection

This part of the assignment involves evaluating the specific cruise options selected using your own criteria. Students should incorporate these criteria in their paper. Criteria can be objective (e.g., time, activities, services) or subjective (e.g., intangible factions such as image, desires, social norms). Be sure to describe the judgments and the information that you used to reach the decision that you made. Be sure to identify the attributes that "pushed" or "pulled" you towards that specific cruise experience. In class we will talk about a wide range of factors that motivate people to make specific travel decisions. Which of the following factors contributed to your decision and how?

- *Physiological* (e.g., escape, relaxation, relief of tension, sun, lust, mental relaxation, release of tension),
- *Safety* (e.g., health, recreation, keep oneself active and healthy for the future),
- *Belonging* (e.g., family togetherness, enhancement of kinship relationships, companionship, facilitation of social interaction, maintenance of personal ties, interpersonal relations, romance or potential for romance),
- *Esteem* (e.g., convince oneself of one's achievements, show ones importance to others, social recognition, ego-enhancement, professional/business, personal development, status and achievement), and
- *Self-actualization* (e.g., exploration and evaluation of self, self-discovery, satisfaction of inner desires).

In other words, this section of your assessment should highlight the dimensions that made each of the cruises an attractive or unattractive option (e.g., what needs pushed you toward the cruise experience and what cruise attributes pulled you toward the specific experience). This section of your assessment should conclude with a short discussion of the factors that may have influenced the ultimate decision that you made relative to the cruise that you actually took (e.g., there might not be transportation available for the cruise you want to take or your friends or families might not be able to take the selected cruise with you or you might really want to go on the party ship, but you are not twenty-one years old).

Purchase and Postpurchase Evaluation

The students should provide a detailed evaluation after the student completes the cruise experience. This section requires the critical examination of the match between expectations for the cruise experience (based on your review of cruise options) and the reality of the experience. This part of the evaluation should focus on those components of the cruise experience that were confirmed and those that were disconfirmed. This section should conclude with an overall evaluation of the student's level of satisfaction or dissatisfaction with the overall cruise experience and why they feel that way. This section should also include recommendations for improving the quality of the cruise experience. This type of an evaluation can be used by owners/managers of the tourist attractions to improve the quality of the tourist experience, to improve operations and effectiveness, and to make decisions about how the operation is doing and how they are affecting the tourists, the community and the environment.

The assessment should include an introduction, a description of all relevant details associated with the cruise experience (type of cruise, when you cruised, who you cruised with, how you traveled to ISSCO, what you did before and after the cruise, etc.), and a summary of what you learned from completing this assignment, and it should be well organized with headings and sub-headings for all relevant sections.

Students are required to complete multiple drafts of each written assignment. A draft of each assignment must be reviewed by a friend or family member. The draft must be signed and dated by the proofreader (include phone number). Reviewers comments should be in red ink and the final version of the assignment should incorporate the comments of the reviewer. The reviewed draft should be submitted to the teaching assistant at the same time the assignment is turned in to Professor Robertson or before the due date of the specific assignment. Failure to submit a peer-reviewed draft will result in a 10% penalty deducted from the final grade on the specific assignment. No exceptions!

24

Class Exercise No. 1

Dr. John Burger

Evolution (Zoology 690)

Introduction

This is the first of two class exercises for which you are responsible during the course of the semester. The general theme of this assignment is the continuing conflict between the teaching of evolutionary biology in the science classroom and creationists. This is an enormously large area of controversy, with strongly-committed protagonists on both sides. Below, you will find a list of suggested topics representing a sampling of different aspects of the controversy. As biologists and citizens, it is important that you have an understanding of the conflict and its background. Some of you will be entering the teaching professions and will be in the "front lines" of the continuing battle between evolution and creationism. This is not a trivial issue. It is deadly serious to many people, including politicians.

Procedures

Summary of Important Dates:

By:	Task:
September 15	Select your topic and submit to JFB
October 11	Complete research, write first draft and submit for peer review
October 18	Complete peer reviews and return to authors
October 25	Submit final draft, first draft and peer review comments to JFB

1. Select a topic for your writing assignment. A sampling of possible topics (by no means an exhaustive list) is given below. Use the Internet to assist you. *Above all*, select a topic about which *you have*

something to say. This is critical to writing a thoughtful paper. I want *Your* perspective on an issue as well as those of others. Please submit your choice of topic in writing to JFB *no later than* September 15. It is important that there be sufficient resources available for your topic and that they be readily accessible to you. Your instructors can assist you in locating resources for your topic.

2. Your written paper should be five to ten single-spaced pages on good quality paper and printed with a good quality laser or ink jet printer. If you require more than ten pages to adequately cover a topic, that is okay but I would prefer not to get any fifty page papers.

3. Sources of information should be cited in the text (author & date) [Jones (1998)], and cited in full in a bibliography at the end of the paper. For Internet sites, cite the author, date, title, and URL (if known). *Do not* use Modern Language Association (MLA) format!

4. *Carefully* follow the guidelines for preparation of your written work. It is critically important that you *read and understand* the guidelines in the handout on "How to Write Clearly, Concisely, and Effectively" for organization and writing style and the handout on "Expectations and Grading Criteria." This writing assignment will count for 20% of your course grade and must not be undertaken lightly! You will be graded on a 100-point scale. Your grade will be based on completeness of coverage, thoughtfulness, clarity of expression, spelling, and good grammar.

5. You can prepare your paper individually, or you can do it with another person (i.e., in pairs). In that case, both students will get the same grade. One advantage of working in pairs is division of labor, especially in researching a topic area.

6. You must submit an initial draft of your work to one of your classmates for peer review *no later than* October 11, but it can be sooner, if you wish. You will receive an initial draft from another classmate to peer review. It is important that you follow the peer review guidelines provided to you so that you can give maximum assistance to your classmates in producing the best possible assignment. Peer reviewers will provide signed written comments on separate sheets for review by the writers. When you receive the peer review of your work, you will respond to the comments in writing. Peer reviews must be returned to authors *no later than* October 18.

7. The final draft of your writing assignment is due on October 25. For every day that your work is late, 10% will be deducted from your grade for the assignment. If your work is 10 days late or more you will receive a "zero" for the assignment. You will submit the following to JFB: (1) first draft of your written work; (2) a copy of peer-review comments; (3) your written responses to peer-review comments; (4) final draft of your work.

8. Feel free to consult JFB for information or resources associated with your topic. He has a large stack of books (most are listed below) and a mountain of articles of all kinds on creationism and evolution. The library is also an excellent source of information as is the internet. An excellent guide to writing is: Jan A. Pechenick. *A Short Guide to Writing About Biology* (especially Chapter 5: revising); 4th edition. A copy is on reserve in the Biological Sciences library, and JFB has a copy.

List of Suggested Topics for Assignment No. 1

1. The "evolution" of creationism from the 1960s to the present time. How has creationist thought changed during that time?

2. The "evolution" of creationist responses to the teaching of evolution in public school science classrooms. How have these responses changed during the past thirty years? What are current strategies for limiting or eliminating the teaching of evolution?

3. "Schools" of creationism in the United States. How do they differ? How are they similar? Which "schools" predominate today? Which ones have the most adherents?

4. Summarize the evidence that contradicts descent with modification and natural selection according to scientists such as Michael Behe (biochemistry and "irreducible complexity") and Phillip Johnson ("Darwin on Trial"), and William Dembski (Dean of the "Intelligent Design" movement) and evaluate its validity.

5. Summarize the evidence for evolution and against creationism as an explanation for the evolution of life on earth and biological diversity as presented by Philip Kitcher ("Abusing Science"), J. William Schopf ("Evolution! Fact and Fallacies"), Douglas Futuyma ("Science on Trial"), Laurie R. Godfrey ("Scientists Confront Creationism") or another author of your choice.

6. Discuss the background of the "Scopes Monkey Trial" (1925) and the events leading up to the trial as well as the effects of the trial

and its aftermath on teaching of evolution in public schools as presented by Edward J. Larsen ("Summer for the Gods").

7. Discuss recent evidence for natural selection in nature. You may need to go to the scientific literature for this. I also have some references. A good start is Jonathan Weiner ("The Beak of the Finch").

8. Discuss the evidence for absolute dating the ages of sediments and the earth by the radiometric method. Include in your discussion different radiometric measures (such as carbon-14 potassium-argon, uranium-lead) and indicate how far back in the past each method can measure. Include in your discussion specific objections by creationists to this method.

9. You teach a high school biology course that includes the concept of evolution. Several of your students have complained to their parents that they are being taught to "believe" in evolution even though they have strong religious objections to godless "Darwinism." Their parents have complained to the principal and the local school board that their children have the right to learn alternatives to evolution and are demanding that you teach alternatives to evolution so the students can learn for themselves what to believe. How do you respond to: (1) the students; (2) the parents; (3) the principal; (4) the local school board? How would you formulate your responses and what resources would you use to explain your position?

10. What is "Creation Science"? How does it differ from "creationism" in general? Is it a valid scientific alternative to "Evolution Science"? Discuss in detail.

11. Discuss the role of the National Center for Science Education (NCSE) in the current debates about teaching evolution and creationist attempts to limit or eliminate the teaching of evolutionary theory in public schools. JFB has NCSE Reports going back several years.

12. Discuss the current status of "Intelligent Design" Creationism, including the role of the Discovery Institute's "Center for the Renewal of Science and Culture" and Jonathan Wells and William Dembski in promoting ID Creationism nationwide.

13. Discuss attempts by various state boards of education and other educational groups to include the teaching or presentation of "alternatives" to evolution, particularly "intelligent design" in public

schools during the past 5-10 years. (NCSE Reports have good summaries of these attempts).

14. Research and summarize the efforts to eliminate, modify or limit the teaching of evolutionary theory in the United States during the past 20 years. Indicate for each state what actions were taken or proposed and the results, including the current status today.

15. Compare and contrast the Arkansas and Louisiana evolution cases. On what basis were court decisions made and what was the impact of these decisions at the time and now?

16. Some people claim that it is "unfair" to present only one point of view when discussing the topic of evolution and arguments against evolution should be presented along side of evidence for evolution so that students can choose what to believe. Discuss both sides of this argument in detail and present your conclusions.

17. Some people with strong religious convictions believe that if evolution is true and that humans are animals just like other animals, then there is no purpose and meaning to human life and this will destroy the moral principles by which human populations live and result in widespread evil and corruption. Is this a valid concern? Does belief in evolution lead to moral decline?

18. Is "Creation Science" science? Is "Creation Science" religion?

19. Discuss in detail the scientific basis for "Creation Science" as outlined by creation scientists. Then evaluate the validity of their theories.

20. Textbook Disclaimers. There have been several states that have required that "disclaimers" be pasted into biology textbooks stating that evolution is "only a theory", and this disclaimer must be read by teachers to their students by state law. Review the content and status of disclaimers in public school textbooks and comment on their relevance to the evolution/creationism debate.

21. To what extent is Creationism in conflict with the teaching of evolutionary theory in other countries? Compare controversies in other countries with those currently in progress in the United States.

22. Outline and discuss the "arguments from design" proposed by "Intelligent Design" (ID) proponents such as Michael Behe and others, and arguments of "irreducible complexity" as a problem for evolutionary biology.

23. Summarize the types of conflicts between proponents of evolutionary biology and Creationists (in the general sense) currently in progress in different states [the news section of NCSE Reports is an excellent source of information as are various web sites].

24. Choose a topic of your own. Find something that interests you! You may wish to consult with JFB about a possible topic to be certain that a specific topic is "doable" and for resources on the topic you have chosen.

25. Discuss the "Wedge Strategy" developed by William Dembski and others in the Intelligent Design movement for replacing evolution with ID ("Creationisms Trojan Horse").

26. Discuss the concept of "fairness" in teaching about "origins" in public school science classes, and attempts by some groups to promote "teaching the controversy" to school and boards and curriculum committees. Is there really a "controversy" about the concepts of evolutionary theory (descent with modification, natural selections, etc.)?

25

Assignment and Group Work Descriptions

Dr. Elizabeth Crepeau

Occupation, Health, and Community Programming (Occupational Therapy 772/872)

Individual Assignments (50%) of course grade)

Community Observation (P/F)

You will observe a public meeting, meeting of a group, or public space. I will provide a list of observation opportunities for the class. This observation should take at least one hour. Each of you will conduct this observation independently and write a report describing your observations. This report should be about three pages in length. Attach any maps or diagrams. Turn in one copy of the report. The report should include the following:

- Location observed: Give location of your observation area, date, and time of your observation. Describe the rooms, buildings, landscape, or other physical features of this area. Are there signs or posters in this area? How does the area "feel" to you? Draw a map or diagram of the location, indicating major physical features and areas where people seem to congregate.
- People: Describe the people you observed, their approximate age (preschool, grade school, young adult, middle age, older adult), gender, etc. Do you have other observations about the people? Locate the people on your map/diagram.
- Activities: What were the people doing as individuals or as groups? List the activities you observed and describe them. Did they interact with each other? How? Did they seem to be enjoying themselves?

Grading: P/F

Grading Criteria:
P: To pass, the observation report must be a clear description of the observation site. It should be so clear that the reader can imagine being there. The actions and affect of the people and the atmosphere of the social and physical environment should be very clear. The report will also be well organized and clearly stated. There will be no obvious errors in grammar, etc.

F: Failing observation reports fail to communicate the scene adequately. Observations are general and lack detail. The reader has a difficult time envisioning the observation site and the people in it. Writing may be less well developed.

Walkability Survey (P/F)

The walkability survey group will be asking each class member to complete a walkability survey of a section of Newmarket. To pass, you must complete the survey within the timeline specified. The survey must be legible and complete. If you can, take photographs of the section of town you are surveying. These may be digital or film, however, digital is the preferred format.

News Flash (P/F)

Each student will present a news flash on a selected week in the semester. This news flash is an informal oral report on a topic related to the class from recent newspapers, magazines, TV or radio reports, or the Internet followed by a brief discussion. The report discussion should not exceed three to five minutes.

Research Summary
(5% of course grade)

Purpose

Your group will be focusing on a task related to enhancing the health of people in Newmarket. The group must real peer-review research methods. Each of you will produce review summaries consisting of a minimum of four related articles. You will use these research summaries as the basis for the literature review. The format of the research summary is on page 23 of this syllabus.

Focus your search on the topic as it relates to your group task. Identify appropriate key words for this topic. In addition to your specific topic, someone in the group should review sources related to habits, behavioral change, motivation, and related topics. The group needs to begin to develop a basic understanding of the strategies that successfully promote lasting behavior change. See the BlackBoard readings section for articles related to habits, behavioral change, motivation, and related topics. You may use a maximum of two articles from BlackBoard for your research summaries.

A research summary is a systematic way of abstracting and organizing research articles. Summaries provide a mechanism to quickly abstract and organize research findings. At the end of the semester you will have a notebook of the research summaries of all class member. You will be able to use this in future courses and during fieldwork and I hope will continue to add to it as you practice occupational therapy.

Assignment

You will be writing four research summaries on a topic related to diabetes, physical activity, obesity, behavioral change/habits, motivation, and/or population-based interventions in occupational therapy. You will draw on recent (typically the past five years) articles in professional journals that either report empirical research or provide a comprehensive review of the literature. See Deci and Ryan (2000) in the Black-Board readings for an example of a comprehensive literature review. The articles you abstract for your individual research summaries will be directly related to your group project. In addition, you will use these summaries for your literature review.

1. Identify the topics your groups should explore for the research summaries. Decide how you would like to divide the work between group members in a way that is equitable. Each group member must search the CDC web site, OT Search, and the diabetes web sites. Divide the UNH online data bases between group members.

2. Each group member must go to the Centers for Disease Control and Prevention web site (www.cdc.gov): This is an excellent website for up-to-date medical and public health research. Develop a strategy in your group for searching this site. There are several parts of the web site that are particularly strong, but you should "noodle" around to see what else you can find. These are very useful parts for your general topic:

- CDC Wonder
- Behavioral Risk Factor Surveillance System
- Health Topics
- Publications: In publications see the Morbidity and Mortality Weekly Report (MWWR), Measuring Health Days, and Physical Activity and Health

3. Use the UNH website for online databases. Go to the health/medicine/sports section of the databases. Check out at least one of the online databases. Particularly helpful databases are PubMed, Psychlit, Sociofile, CINAHL, Web of Science. Divide the web sites between group members. Each group member should search one web site for the topics of other group members.

4. Find out what the occupational therapy literature has to say about population-based programming and prevention programs and behavioral change/motivation. OT Search is included in the UNH online databases. Explore OT Search to see what resources are available on it. It has some significant strengths—but also some significant limitations!

5. Find out what the American Diabetes Association and other professional associations have to say about diabetes prevention and public education. See the ADA at www.diabetes.org and their journal at www.diabetesjournal.org. (Note: this latter web site will gain you access to current diabetes literature. You may purchase articles from the web site (an expensive decision) or request interlibrary loan for those journals not carried by the UNH library. Note: Interlibrary loan typically takes seven to ten days to deliver an article.

6. For each search print out the search result with full citations and abstract. Aim to have at least five articles from each web site/source you have searched. In class, meet with group members and share what you have found. Divide the articles among group members so that each member has four articles on the topic for his or her literature review.

Grading Criteria

A: To achieve this grade, your summary must be complete and clearly written. Enough information is abstracted so that the reader is able to assess the value of the research and its contribution to the understanding of the topic. To the extent possible, write this summary in your own words, however, you may quote directly if necessary. No typographical errors, APA is correct, etc.

B: A "B" matrix falls short of the "A" criteria in that the research is either not abstracted clearly enough to fully understand the methods and findings or is too detailed to "qualify" as an abstract. No typographical errors, APA is correct, etc.

C: A "C" matrix is difficult to understand or incomplete. The reader is left wondering what the research is about or why the findings would be important. There may be typographical or APA errors.

F: An "F" matrix reflects a complete lack of understanding of the research being abstracted. The reader is left wondering what the research is about and why the findings would be important. There may be typographical and APA errors.

Literature Review (15% individual)

Purpose

The purpose of this assignment is to learn how to synthesize findings from a *minimum of five related articles (empirical articles/comprehensive literature reviews) that address a focused topic.* Each literature review will form a "chapter" in the final report of the group. Consequently, each literature review must address a separate but related aspect of the groups' topic.

Description of a literature review

A literature review synthesizes and discusses the empirical research regarding a focused topic. Your paper should describe the current best thinking on your topic. It should not be just a recitation of the individual research articles, but a synthesis of them. It should be written in your own words (e.g., do not use direct quotations) and should be cited using the APA format. The paper should be between three and five pages, excluding title page and reference list.

Here are some ways to think about your paper:
- What is the current understanding of X? (e.g., the dangers of obesity in children)
- What is the influence of X or Y? (e.g., walking on blood pressure)
- What are the causes of X? (e.g., type II diabetes, children not walking to school)

Time Line:

_____   Meet with your groups to decide on the topics for each of your papers.

_____   Share these topics with the entire class so that others can suggest resources for you.

_____   Gather resources, read the articles, and bring them to class. Be prepared to begin writing in class. I will save thirty minutes in class for you to get started.

_____   Peer review papers. If you would like me to review a draft of your paper, you should revise it and turn it in to me by the date specified.

_____   Turn in completed literature review.

_____   Review literature review after it is graded for inclusion in the final report of your group.

Grading Criteria

A papers: An A paper is concise and clear. The student has utilized excellent sources (up-to-date empirical research or literature reviews from high-quality professional journals). The research findings are clearly presented in the words of the student. The research findings are synthesized, that is each study is not reported independently, rather the findings of all papers are discussed in an integrated way. By the end of the paper, the reader has a clear understanding of the research related to the topic, its strengths, its weaknesses, and issues for future research. The APA format is carefully followed for in-text citation and the reference list.

B papers: B papers adequately address the topic. The student has utilized excellent sources (up-to-date empirical research or literature reviews from high quality professional journals). The reader can tell the student has a grasp of the research. However, the research may not be adequately synthesized. There may be some direct quotations and minor problems with organization, development of ideas, and clarity in English. These my interrupt the flow of the paper or lead to areas of confusion. There may be very minor problems with citation of sources in the text or on the reference list.

C papers: C papers address the topic; however, there are significant weaknesses in the development of the ideas and the clarity of writing. The sources may not be of excellent quality or may not be peer-reviewed empirical research or literature reviews published in professional journals. The student displays a limited understanding of the topic. There may be very minor problems with citation of sources in the text or on the reference list.

F paper. F papers address the topic; however, there are significant weaknesses in the development of the ideas and the clarity of writing. Sources may not be of excellent quality or may not be peer-reviewed empirical research or literature reviews published in professional journals. It is clear that the student did not understand the material sufficiently to explain it in writing. There are problems with citation of sources in the text or on the reference list.

Health Fair Presentation/Demonstration/Poster (10% of course grade)

Purpose

One of the goals of this course is to have you develop an appreciation for the role occupational therapists can play in fostering the health of the community. Health fairs are one way to educate community members about health issues.

Assignment

You will develop a presentation/demonstration/poster related to your group project for the Health Fair in Newmarket. This presentation will be peer reviewed by your classmates.

Grading

A: An A presentation/poster/demonstration will be entertaining and informative. health information will be correct and stated in language appropriate for audience. All printed materials or demonstration items will be well-developed, clear, and professional in appearance. The student will be confident in demeanor and will answer questions clearly and in language appropriate for the audience.

B: A B presentation/poster/demonstration will have sufficient information, but will contain language at a level that is not appropriate for the audience. Information may not be clearly presented and may be "boring."

C: A C demonstration/poster/presentation will have insufficient information, etc.

F: A F demonstration/poster/presentation will demonstrate that the writer has an incomplete understanding of the research and therefore cannot communicate it effectively.

Goal Attainment Paper (20% of course grade)

One aspect of this course is to articulate professional development and healthy lifestyle goals. These goals will be in behavioral form (observable, measurable)

You will write two goals for the course. One goal will target your professional development. This goal may addresses the development of oral and written communication skills, assertiveness, responsibility to group members, or any other goal that you feel will enhance your development as a future occupational therapist. The second goal will address a personal health goal. Examples of goals may include:

- I will contribute to class discussions by sharing my ideas, making suggestions, and/or answering questions. I will speak at least one time in each class and will keep a tally of these contributions that records my specific contributions and my affective response to making them.
- I will fulfill my responsibility to group members by being on time for all group meetings, notifying the group if I will be late or absent, and completing my tasks on time and with a high level of competence.
- I will increase the frequency of attending aerobics classes from three times a week to four.
- I will begin an exercise program by walking 10,000 steps a day as measured by a pedometer.

Remember, you should develop goals that are reasonable for you to attain within the context of this course and your "life" in general. *Be realistic in articulating your goals.*

Because the goals you articulate represent your aspirations for change across the semester, we will break these down into a short term action plan. This plan will be reassessed every two weeks. You will write a final paper that articulates both what you have achieved relative to your objectives for the semester and your insights about this process relative to your future role as an occupational therapist.

Paper

Purpose

This is an integrative paper that links your experience with your goal attainment this semester and your thoughts about goal setting as part of occupational therapy practice with pertinent readings from the semester. You are not expected to do additional research/reading for this paper beyond what you have already read in the course. Please address the following.

About You: Analyze your goal achievement this semester. How successful were you in achieving your goals? What contributed to this success? What barriers to goal achievement did you encounter and how did you attempt to overcome them? What have you learned about yourself during this process? Link your answer to EHP, explaining the theory of your experience in the context of this theoretical perspective. Be explicit about the relationship between the theory and your experience. How does this theory help you understand and explain your experience?

About behavioral change: What have you learned about behavioral change? Link your observations to the material you have learned in this class and your group project. Cite specific readings demonstrating your understanding of the relationship between the empirical research and your experience. Include the contribution of EHP and the research about behavioral change, motivation, etc. Be sure to explain the theoretical perspective adequately to convey your understanding of them and your ability to apply them

About your future clients: How will the process of setting goals we used this semester inform your OT practices? Address specifically the goal setting process. How has this assignment helped you think about your future clients as individuals embedded in their unique context? In what way did this assignment help you think about clients from a more occupation-based, client-centered perspective?

This paper should not exceed six to eight pages, excluding cover page and reference list.

Grading

I will base your grade for this assignment on the degree to which your analysis indicates your understanding of the theoretical material presented in the course, and your ability to apply this information to your experiences this semester and your future practice as an occupational therapist.

A papers: An A paper is comprehensive and addresses all of the questions in the assignment. It is very clearly written and cited. Pertinent research is clearly described in the student's words. The paper reflects an excellent understanding of the concepts of EHP, motivation, behavioral change, etc. and the ability to apply this theoretical information to the student's experience, behavior change, and future clients. APA citations are correct.

B papers: B papers are similar to A papers except that they either lack clarity or do not adequately link research and concepts from EHP to the questions. Writing is generally competent. APA citations are correct.

C papers: C papers lack both clarity and information. It is not clear that the student understands the material sufficiently to apply it or communicate it to others. Writing may have organizational problems and is confusing to the reader. There may be problems with APA citations.

F papers: F papers are deficient in information and analysis. Theoretical material is inadequately described. Little or no attempt is made to apply the theoretical perspectives to the goal exercise or future OT practice. Problems with APA citations.

Working Groups (30% of final grade)

This semester the class has six major tasks to accomplish. I will be asking you for your preferences regarding which tasks you prefer. One the basis of your preferences, I will form the groups. The talks involve both primary prevention and secondary prevention activities. The tasks are as follows:

I.   **Diabetes Self-Management Program Development (Secondary Prevention):** Type II diabetes is a chronic illness that requires careful dietary management, physical exercise, blood sugar monitoring, and medication management to prevent the onset of complications secondary to the disease. These complications include heart attack, stroke, kidney disease, diabetic retinopathy, and diabetic neuropathy. Lamprey Health Care has a comprehensive diabetes program; however, they would like to improve their services to their patients with diabetes. Your role will be to assist them in this process.

1. Review the work of the previous group and the Lamprey diabetes self-management materials (this includes the material from the collaborative, the Bayer material, plus anything else you want the students to review.

2. Develop new, modify existing, or recommend existing self-management programs for use at Lamprey Health Care. This program should be client-centered and occupation-based. This program will include goals for the program and will delineate a plan for each meeting including specific objectives, activities, handouts, evaluation procedures.

3. Obtain approval of this curriculum from Lamprey Health Care. Implement the self-management program at Lamprey.

4. Make an oral presentation (including power point slides) to the nurse/provider meeting in Newmarket.

   Final Report: This report will include the self-management program curriculum and an analysis of its implementation, including recommendations for modification for future groups. this report will cite pertinent research literature and will be written in a style consistent with the APA format.

II. **Recreation Department Walking Program (primary prevention):** Last fall a group developed the Recreation Department Walking Program. The participants enjoyed the program and would like to continue it. Your group will be focusing on evaluating and maintaining the walking group at the Recreation Department.

1. Conduct a focus group of the women who participated in the Recreation Center Walking Program last fall. The purpose of this focus group is to evaluate the effectiveness of the program and the facilitators and barriers to continuing the program over the winter.

2. Based on the findings of the focus group, if needed, adapt the walking program by id-February. This adaptation will directly address barriers to walking identified by the group, for example winter weather and the closed campus in the summer.

3. Develop a schedule for the walking program and organize the class so that all class members walk at least once during the semester.

4. Design and implement an evaluation to assess the effectiveness of the walking program relative to health outcomes and satisfaction.

5. Make an oral presentation to Recreation Department personnel and walking program participants in November.

   Final Report: The final report will consist of a synthesis of the focus groups and interviews, the walking group protocol for the Recreation Department, the evaluation and findings. The report will cite pertinent research literature and will be in a style consistent with the APA format.

III. **Lamprey Health Care Employee Walking Program (primary prevention):** In spring 2003 and 2004 a group of students initiated an employee walking program at Lamprey Health Care. Although people were enthusiastic about the program, participation lagged during the eight weeks it occurred. Last fall, the group designed a pedometer program that was successful with some of the employees at Lamprey. They are interested in continuing to develop this program.

1. Review the literature regarding employee-sponsored walking programs (most likely focusing on pedometer programs) and the research that examines the effectiveness of these programs—see the report from last fall's group to get you started.

2. Review the literature on motivation, incentives in employee walking programs, and use of electronic media to support exercise programs.

3. Based on your literature review, design a BB supported mechanism for pedometer walking program participants.

4. Develop an evaluation to assess the effectiveness of the program.

5. Make an oral presentation (power point) to the senior management team.

   Final Report: The final report will consist of a synthesis of the protocol for the walking program, the use of electronic media to support walkers, and the program evaluation. The report will cite pertinent research literature and will be in a style consistent with the APA format.

IV. **Walking School Bus: Newmarket Elementary School (primary prevention):** Today most children ride the school bus or are driven to school by one of their parents. In addition, many children get little physical activity after school because of safety concerns in their neighborhood or the enticements of TV and computer games.

1. Review the work students conducted in the fall, contact interested parents, and plan a walking school bus program for one neighborhood.

2. Propose this program to the school board and parents. Gain approval to initiate the walking school bus from the school board.

3. Implement the walking school bus.

4. Prepare a presentation (power point) on the walk-to-school program for the PTO or another appropriate group.

   Final Report: The group will write a paper that synthesizes their work with the research literature. The report will be written in a style consistent with the APA format.

V. **Recess Program for fourth- and fifth-graders at Newmarket Elementary School:** Today most children ride the school bus or are driven to school by one of their parents. In addition, many children get little physical activity after school because of safety concerns in their neighborhood or the enticements of TV and computer games. The recess program will focus on the development of activities that the children enjoy that will enhance their physical activity.

1. Develop a recess program aimed to increase physical activity and life style changes for twenty-four fourth- and fifth-graders on Tuesdays and Thursdays from 11:30 to 12:20. The program will run from approximately mid-February through the last week of classes.

2. Gain approval of the program from appropriate school personnel.

3. Implement the program on February 8th (note the students are on Winter break the week of February 21 and Spring Break the week of April 25th).

4. Once the program is established, recruit classmates to assist with the activities. (Everyone in the class should participate, but I expect your group members to take the responsibility for planning and leading each session.)

5. Develop and implement an assessment to identify the effectiveness of the program.

6. Prepare a presentation (power point) for the PTO, school board, or other appropriate group.

Final Report: The group will write a paper that synthesizes their work with the research literature. The report will be written in a style consistent with the APA format.

VI. **Walkability Survey Group (primary prevention):** Last spring students began a walkability survey of the town of Newmarket. They focused on the downtown streets. Your group will be responsible to continue this process focusing on surveying another area of town. Your group has the following tasks:

1. Review the work of the previous group and the materials from the Livable Walkable Community websites and plan the walkability survey of the section of Newmarket assigned to your group.

2. Divide the survey among group members asking for assistance from classmates. (Everyone in the class should participate, but I expect your group members to do a greater proportion of the surveying).

3. Describe the survey results street by street summarizing the questions from the survey (a chart might be the best way to do this).

4. Record survey results on the town maps indicating walking conditions by criteria on the walkability survey (how does your neighborhood stack up?).

5. Make recommendations for the town planner regarding changes needed to increase the walkability of the streets surveyed. Indicate which areas have the highest priority from your perspective.

6. Prepare an oral report for the Town Council Workshop.

    Final Report: Your final report should include a summary of the survey results and maps, recommendations for the town, and pertinent research literature.

    Final Report Format: This is the general format for the final paper. The specifics of each group report will vary; however, the format should be relatively consistent group to group. The group reports from previous semesters should not be used as this assignment has evolved from the initial offering of this course. Please include the following:

    • Title Page

    • Table of Contents

- Introduction: The introduction should describe your task and lead the reader through the rest of the paper. Provide an introduction to the literature base for your task.

- Chapters 1-5 (or whatever number of members you have in your group): These chapters are the literature reviews that you wrote individually. The reference lists should be combined at the end of the report. Each group member should revise his or her literature review based on the feedback given when the review was graded earlier in the semester. In addition, feedback from other group members should be used to review these chapters.

- Chapter 6: Describe your project, the task and what you accomplished. What did you discover (for example if you conducted interviews, what did your interviewees say). The nature of each project report will vary depending upon the group task. Include a discussion of the discussion from your presentation, if there was significant discussion. This chapter may be divided into multiple chapters.

- Chapter 7: This chapter should include recommendations for future groups who will build on your work. Include strategies that you used that worked, plus problems you encountered and how you solved or didn't resolve them. Recommend the next steps for this project if you feel the project should be continued by students in the future.

- Reference List: Include all references used in the report using APA citation conventions.

- Appendices (put in an order that makes sense—again the contents of the appendices will vary dependent upon your group task)

  - Public affairs announcements—combine these in a single file (only the uncited versions)

  - Power point presentation—one slide/page

  - Interview schedule/focus group schedule

  - IRB (if your group task requires one)

- Resource List for students: Include names, addressed, phone numbers, email addresses and any other information students continuing the project might find useful.

Discuss with your group how you will draft, revise, and edit this document. You should not plan to work as a group-of-the-whole in completing this report; rather, people should divide the responsibilities among group members. We will discuss ways of doing this at about mid-semester.

Midterm Feedback: At midterm you will complete a self-assessment and assessment of group members. These assessments will be shared with your group members. This is a structured opportunity for you to give feedback to your group members regarding the collaborative efforts of the group and the level of cooperation and commitment exhibited by group members.

End of Semester Grading: I will grade this report using criteria consistent with the criteria listed for other assignments. Group members will rate themselves and their group peers on their level of effort for the entire semester. I will average these ratings and weight the final report grade according to the average rating of the group members. For example, if the group report was of A quality, but one group member was rated at 75% effort, this person's grade would be adjusted by this percentage.

Contribution to Collective Learning (5% of course grade)

There are a number of class activities that reflect your contribution to the collective learning of the class and to the various projects. One of these is your presence at meetings/events that will occur outside of class. You are also expected to assist other groups in the implementation of their projects. These responsibilities will be delineated/announced during the semester. Completion of pass/fail assignments will be considered part of this grade. Also, class members will have the opportunity to nominate three classmates who have contributed to the learning of the entire class. These nominations will also contribute to this part of the grade for the course.

A: Participation in the course is marked by active participation in class discussions, completing all pass/fail assignments on time, going above and beyond in helping other groups by walking, helping out with recess programs, etc. Receives a minimum of three nominees by peers.

B: Performance at B level meets the expectations of the class. This person contributes to class discussions, but not frequently. He or she helps by walking, etc. but may do only the minimum expected. Receives no more than two peer nominations.

C: Performance at the C level reflects minimum oral participation in class and in projects beyond the student's immediate group. Pass/fail assignments completed. No peer nominations.

F: Performance at F level reflects minimal involvement in class, pass/fail assignments may not be completed, no peer nominations.

26 Syllabus and Assignment Descriptions

Dr. Michael Kalinowski

International Approaches to Child Advocacy (Family Studies 772)

This course is designed to introduce students to child advocacy. It is a demanding, senior/graduate level elective course that will require significant reading and preparation time and some experiences outside normal class meeting times. Students will analyze readings, review policies, share information, and write papers, with an emphasis on improving one's analytical and communicative skills. This course will be taught similar to a graduate seminar, with students taking increasing responsibility for substantive class contributions.

Over the semester we will review the need for child advocacy, historical issues, exemplary advocates, individual vs. collective advocacy, case and class advocacy, legislative and judicial and executive advocacy, the role of specialized agencies, effective strategies, and selected national and international issues. For Family Studies majors—Prerequisites: FS 525, 645. Recommended: FS 623.

The amount of reading required for class, consistent with other senior level courses, will be significantly greater than that generally assigned in 500 and 600 level courses. We will develop initial required readings over the first several weeks.

Texts

Edelman, Marian Wright. (1992). *The Measure of Our Success*. Boston, MA: Beacon Press.

Clinton, Hillary Rodham. (1996). *It Takes a Village*. New York, NY: Simon & Schuster.

APA. (2001). *Publication Manual of the American Psychological Association.* Fifth edition.

Computers

Computer literacy is an essential skill for advocates; all work submitted must be completed on a computer. Students without previous computer experience or who have computer anxiety may receive assistance upon request, but should ask for help early in the course. Students will work with the Internet, ERIC, UNH library and other databases and search engines. Students must inform the instructor within the first two classes if they are not familiar with computers. All students must submit an email address to the instructor.

Assignments

There are five graded activities in this course.

Participation

This class process may be somewhat different from what you may be accustomed to in typical lecture courses. Child advocates must be prepared to take active positions on behalf of children and be held accountable for them. Students are expected to come to class prepared, having completed all assigned readings and ready to contribute to the day's discussion. A significant portion of your grade will be based on class participation, as evidenced by your attendance, regular class contributions, integration of material from readings and discussions and lectures, ability to consider the perspective of others, willingness to take action and defend a position, and attempts to search for innovative solutions. Over the course of the semester, a student may "buy a vowel" (pass on a question) once if the student feels unprepared. If anyone ever feels more than momentarily uncomfortable at the participation requirement, please speak to the instructor immediately.

Field Trip Day

Students should expect to spend one Friday (7:30-3:30 TBA) observing exemplary child advocacy programs, attending advocacy information sessions, and/or visiting experts. After this trip, students will complete a brief reaction paper. This is not an activity that can be made up. One class will be cancelled to take into account time allocated to these field trips.

Short Papers

Students will complete several brief (one- to three-page) papers reacting to cases, comparing experiences to those described in their readings, and planning advocacy strategies.

Position Papers

Students will write a position paper (twelve pages) analyzing one significant child advocacy issue, including a comparison between that issue in the United States and another (non-English-speaking) country. This will require time throughout the semester gathering print and internet sources, studying the issues, obtaining information from your selected country, and preparing and revising drafts.

Quizzes/Reflections

There will be a handful of (usually unannounced) quizzes or requests for students to reflect on their readings or materials covered in class.

Evaluation

Participation	25 points
Field Trip	10 points
Short papers (3 @ 5 points)	15 points
Position Paper	30 points
Quizzes/Reflections (5 @ 4 points)	20 points
Total	100 points

Course Policies

Academic Integrity

Violating academic integrity is considered a serious offense by the university and is treated accordingly. Violation of academic integrity includes, but is not limited to, all of the following: cheating on exams, having unauthorized possession of exams, and submitting the work of another person as your own (plagiarism). Academic dishonesty may result in a failing grade for the particular assignment or exam, a failing grade for the entire course, or suspension or expulsion from the university. Please consult the current version of the UNH *Students' Rights, Rules, and Responsibilities*.

APA Style

Please use APA style for all of your work. Students may fail an assignment if appropriate APA style is not utilized.

Deadlines

Deadlines help students (and faculty) organize their workloads and enable the instructor to treat students equitably. A student's grade on any assignment will be reduced by one grade for each day or portion of a day an assignment is late. In very rare occasions a brief extension might be considered before the deadline for a student with a death in the family, major accident, etc. In such cases documentation will be required. No extensions will be granted after a deadline.

Disability Accommodations

If you need disability accommodations, please contact UNH ACCESS, Support Services for Students with Disabilities, located in 118 Memorial Union Building, (603) 862-2607 as soon as possible. All information regarding disabilities is confidential, and I will be pleased to cooperate with Access to make necessary accommodations.

Participation in University Events

Students who miss class due to participation in university-sanctioned activities must identify themselves prior to missing class and make arrangements to complete missing work.

Nonsexist Language

The UNH Policy on Nonsexist Language requires that all written and oral communications be free from sex-biased terminology. Please keep this in mind when completing your assignments and let me know about any errors that I may make in this regard. Thanks.

Support for Written Assignments

This course is an approved Writing Intensive (WI) course and demands considerable writing, reflection, and revision. Please consult each other, with the graduate students, and with the Writing Center as well as with me.

Major Paper

Overview

Students will write a position paper (12 pages) analyzing one significant child advocacy issue, including a comparison between that issue in the United States and another (non-English-speaking) country. This will require time throughout the semester gathering print and internet sources, studying the issues, obtaining information from your selected country, and preparing and revising drafts. I do not want to read your first or second draft.

Length

Minimum of 12 pages.

Deadlines

A draft of the paper is due no later than 12:00 noon on Wednesday, November 23. The final, revised paper must be submitted to my office no later than 6:10 p.m. on Friday, December 9.

Points

Up to 30 points may be earned for this assignment.

Suggested Format

The following format is required. Minimum requirements for the length of each section are listed under "Pages." The last date a Draft and Final version can be accepted is also noted. Sections with asterisk are those considered the most important. Dates in **bold** indicate there is no class that day.

Pages	Chapter	Draft	Final
—	Abstract	12/2	**12/9**
1	Intro, definition, and issue in form of a question	**11/23**	**12/9**
5	Review of the Literature in America*	**11/23**	**12/9**
4	Review of the Literature in Chosen Country*	**11/23**	**12/9**
2	Recommend Actions*	**11/23**	**12/9**
0.5	Personal Observations	**11/23**	**12/9**
—	References	**11/23**	**12/9**

References

Students are expected to utilize a *minimum* of ten sources, in the most appropriate combination of print, Internet, media, correspondence, and interview references. Most will use more.

Style

The manuscript must follow APA style, and must not have NOS or ROS.

Abstracts

"An abstract is a brief, comprehensive summary of the contents of [a paper]; it allows readers to survey the contents of an article quickly and, like a title, it enables abstracting and information services to index and retrieve articles . . . A well prepared abstract can be the most important paragraph in your article" (APA, 2001, p. 12).

Start by reading the APA section [1.07] on abstracts. Then look at abstracts at the beginning of research articles you uncover for examples.

According to the APA (2001, pg. 12), a "good abstract is

1. **accurate**: Write the abstract to reflect your purpose and content. Compare your draft with your outline (headings and subheadings).

2. **self-contained**: Define abbreviations when first used. Define unique terms. Do not quote, paraphrase when necessary. If essential, cite author(s) and dates if you need to cite a publication. Include 3-7 keywords (in boldface) within the abstract for indexing.

3. **concise and specific**: Be brief. Do not exceed 960 characters and spaces, or about 120. Start with the most important information. Do not repeat title. Include only the most relevant findings.

4. **non-evaluative**: Report. Do not add to or comment on your paper.

5. **coherent & readable**: Write in the present tense. Use the third person. Use active verbs rather than nouns. Do not waste words or nonessential sentences."

Your abstract should use this format:

1. State the problem being investigated in one sentence.

2. Note both the United States and your other country in that first sentence.

3. Introduce your major discoveries in one or two sentences for each country.

4. Very briefly summarize the most compelling comparison between the issue in your country and the United States.

5. Briefly note your top two recommended actions.

6. You should expect to write *at least* three drafts; writing abstracts is hard because of the limitations. I will try to review your draft very quickly.

27

Laboratory Instructions

Dr. Barry Fussell

Experimental Measurement and Data Analysis (Mechanical Engineering 646)

Pre-Lab

The lab writeup should be thoroughly read and an outline of the necessary procedures and data needed should be developed. Often some prelab calculations or models will greatly enhance your ability to finish the lab in a timely fashion. You are responsible to take enough data while in the lab to answer all questions asked.

Lab Journal

Each student is required to keep a written lab journal record (**bound or spiral ring**) of their work during the laboratory class. The journal will be briefly reviewed by the lab TAs before the student leaves the lab (worth five points of the lab report). A short, but complete, lab report (**separate from the journal**) is to be turned in one week after class. I am looking for a **concise** and **cohesive** lab report that gives the results, explains them, and answers all lab questions. All reports are to be typed.

You can work with your lab partners on the lab reports in developing plots, tables, data, etc. However, the discussion of the results must be your own work!

Required contents of the lab journal are described below:

1. The date the lab was performed.

2. Identification of the experiment by title.

3. Your name and the names of the other students in your group.

4. List of equipment used in the lab, and a *sketch of the lab setup*.

5. Original data in tabular form.

6. Rough calculations where appropriate. (Formula and sources are to be given in the lab report)

7. Notes on changes in procedure, difficulties encountered and the method used to overcome these difficulties.

Note that a full record of the lab work should be kept it the journal, including any "scratch" work. Thus, it would be prudent to keep your organized results on the front pages of the bound lab notebook, and your scratch work on the backsides. The scratch work will not be reviewed in any way, so it provides you room to keep unorganized information.

Lab Reports

Lab writeups should follow the suggested organization for an **internal engineering report** or some abbreviated form as described below.

Short Engineering Report

Shorten the internal report form by excluding the table of contents and equipment tested, and by using the same organization as the lab handout to give results. Just answer the lab questions and give a brief discussion when appropriate. This lab report is to be short!

External Engineering Report

Follow the internal report except you should include a transmittal letter, cover, and a list of figures as described in Chapter 6 of *A Guide to Writing as an Engineer*, by Beer and McMurrey, John Wiley and Sons, 1997. **You should have this book.** Also, please refer to this book for tips to make your writing more concise, informative, and fun to read!

For the **group short engineering report,** just follow the given shortened form and hand in **one lab report per lab group.**

For the **group internal and external engineering reports,** follow the given form as a group, except for the discussion section, where each student is to write their own section and include it in the report. That is, hand in **one report** for the group containing separate **discussion sections for each individual** of the group. Make sure each discussion is labeled with the appropriate student name, and make sure it is original with no plagiarism. Discussions that contain near verbatim sentences will get zero points! **This is an individual effort!**

28

Paper Topics

Dr. Steven Trzaskoma

Major Greek Authors in English (Classics 421)

Possible Paper Topics for Two- to Three-Page Papers

Topic 1: It was said in antiquity by Xenophon and others (and has been said in modern times) that Socrates courted condemnation and death at his trial by giving a speech designed to provoke the jurors. Assuming (big assumption . . . but let's stick with it) that Plato's *Apology* is a relatively accurate account of Socrates' defense speech, approach this question: Did Socrates truly defend himself as well as he could?

Topic 2: Does Socrates in the *Apology* adequately answer his "old accusers," i.e., the picture painted of him in Aristophanes' *Clouds*?

Topic 3: Read Xenophon's (significantly shorter) *Apology*, which is also in your *Trials of Socrates* book (pp. 177-184). Compare it in some way to Plato's.

Topic 4: What is the ultimate message that Aristophanes intended his audience to take away from the *Clouds*?

Topic 5: A few moderns have asserted that Aristophanes' burlesque of Socrates in the *Clouds* is not intended to be serious. Instead, this line of reasoning goes, the true target of the comedy are the Athenians themselves, as represented by Strepsiades. I'll tell you right up front—I don't buy it. But if you can come anywhere near proving it, I'll be impressed.

Topic 6: How are we to interpret Alcibiades' role in the *Symposium*? Why does Plato have him burst into the party? How does what he says support (or not) Socrates' (and Diotima's) ideas?

Topic 7: Jason as Sophist. Go.

Section 4

Writing Guides
from across the Disciplines

29

Guide for Papers

Dr. John Ernest

English

Part 1: Evaluation

I will evaluate your performance in three basic categories of concern: structure, content, and presentation. Each category will count for approximately one-third of your grade for the paper—though, of course, poor performance in one category inevitably will affect the success of the others. That is, don't assume that I can or will "just read for the ideas" in a poorly presented or illogically constructed essay. I am particularly dismayed when I see errors that are repeated from essay to essay, so make a special effort to apply criticisms of earlier essays to later writing assignments in the class.

I've indicated throughout this guide my standards for evaluation, but I will summarize a few points here, which I've borrowed from similar summaries from other professors.

An "A" Essay

1. has a clearly indicated thesis (or working hypothesis) to which all elements of the essay are relevant;

2. has focused topic sentences that announce the central argument of each paragraph, connecting this new stage of the analysis to that of the previous paragraph;

3. supports its argumentative claim with evidence from the text, and avoids being simply mechanical in citing evidence;

4. attends to the implications of the central argument;

5. is thoughtful and deliberate in its use of language, essay structure, and evidence;

6. considers, if only implicitly, the evidence and arguments that might undermine or challenge the essay's argument, and doesn't ignore important evidence or complications;

7. is free of recurring surface errors or errors of fact;

8. is professional in its presentation—including the title of the essay, page numbers, works-cited format, and other issues of manuscript form;

9. makes no unsupported claims about history, and demonstrates that the essay's author is aware of larger cultural and ideological forces that might distort her or his judgment;

10. is equally attentive to detail and to the big picture;

11. is compelling in its intellectual and ethical commitment to the essay's subject.

Here is another way to think about these concerns—this time with greater emphasis on your responsibilities as a scholar:

- **focus.** You should narrow down your concerns to a reasonably focused set of questions and/or concerns, and use the essay to explore those concerns.

- **specificity.** You should be as specific as you can about the questions you have. If you have questions about African American religion, for example, you should focus on specific historical periods, specific situations, and perhaps even specific denominations or manifestations of religion. If you have questions about the system of slavery, push yourself to look beyond the abstract level and at specific issues within the system.

- **literary skill.** You should include in your paper a discussion of at least one (and, depending on the length and complexity of the work, perhaps more) work of literature. We are reading literature as part of our effort to "read" U.S. history and culture. Present examples of literature that pertain to questions you raise about history and culture, and think about how the author's handling of the work of literature provides insights into, for example, how to interpret the workings of culture.

- **use of information.** The various texts we are reading provide a great deal of useful information. I expect you to make use of this information in your papers. Moreover, when you raise questions that can be answered by a quick look at an encyclopedia (especially specialized ones like the Encyclopedia of African American Culture and History), I expect you to look at that encyclopedia. In other words, I expect you to do basic research on matters of simple information (people and events in history, for example)

- **complexity.** These papers should be challenging, for we are reading about and discussing challenging issues. I expect to encounter a certain intensity of thought in your essays, and I will be critical of any tendency to simplify the issues.
- **grammar and style.** Your writing should be clear and correct, and I should be able to follow your line of thought without using a map.
- **presentation.** Remember to cite your sources, both in the body of the essay and in the bibliography or "works cited" page. For English essays, scholars general use the Modern Language Association (MLA) or the Chicago format for citing sources—and handbooks on both are available in the library. A short sample of proper citations is included at the end of this guide.

Part 2: Manuscript Form and Presentation (and Other Important Details)

Your paper must meet the grammatical and formal standards of academic prose. Leave yourself time to revise, and revise with a grammar handbook close by. Type carefully, and double-space the lines. For conventions concerning the proper handling of quotations, the presentation of titles of works, and the documentation of sources, see the *MLA Handbook for Writers of Research Papers*. A copy is available at the Reference department of Dimond Library. If you are an English major and do not yet own a copy of this book, buy one.

Remember also that academic conventions of clarity and formality are important. Avoid hazy generalizations and other forms of vagueness. A good way to check for this problem is to look at the main verbs and nouns in your sentences: do they tend to be abstract and general, or specific? If the former, change the noun or verb to something more specific rather than adding adjectives or adverbs. One source of ambiguity can be pronouns: make sure that your reader clearly knows what "this" and "that" refer to or, better yet, include clarifying nouns along with the pronouns ("this idea," "that action"). "This" or "that" should not be the subject of any sentence in your essay.

Avoid also cliches, jargon, reductive expressions, and hollow modifiers like "interesting," "positive," "negative," or "successful." Please use gender-neutral language: he or she, hers or his, etc. Remember that there is nothing that warms a professor's heart so much as the carefully, memorably turned phrase or well-written passage. Good writing simply gives your argument more authority and weight and demonstrates your care as a scholar (as well as stylist). All the elements that make for good creative writing also make for good academic writing, so show some creativity and care in your prose. Working within the formal conventions of academic writing does not need to be restrictive; working with and against those conventions—fulfilling them, following the rules (and knowing when, how, and why to break the rules at times), while also speaking with an individual voice—can be a very creative process.

You are required to follow MLA format for citing your sources. I have used this format in this guide so that you will have a model to follow. At the end of this guide is a sample "Works Cited" page.

The following are special instructions or reminders—which means that ignoring them might have a special effect on your grade. **If you do not follow these guidelines concerning spacing, citation, and/or page numbering, then the best grade you can get on your paper is an "A-."**

1. Your essay must be typed, and double-spaced. You should have standard 1-inch margins on the top, bottom, and sides.

2. Note the proper form of parenthetical citation demonstrated in this guide. Remember to indent long quotations. Remember also to provide page numbers for all quotations.

3. Your essay should have a title. An intriguing title can actually add to the power of an argument.

4. Number the pages of your paper (upper right-hand corner; include your last name).

5. Please do not present your paper in a plastic cover. Simply staple the pages once, on the upper left-hand corner. If you are using continuous-feed computer paper, you should of course separate the sheets.

6. Keep a copy of your paper. I've never lost a paper, but you are required keep a copy just in case. Even if I lose your paper, you are still responsible for it.

7. **Proofread your paper before you submit it.** Correct errors before you hand in the paper. If you spot some at the last minute, when it is too late to print a new copy of the paper, please correct the errors neatly with a pen. Spelling and grammar count.

8. If you are using ellipsis points, leave a space between the points:
    Bad, very bad: ...
    Good, very good: . . .

9. Use two hyphens to form a dash, and leave no space between the end of the previous word and the beginning of the dash—so that it will look like this one when you print it.

10. Use brackets when you insert something into or change something in a quotation.
    example: At first, Douglass seems optimistic, for his "new mistress [proves] to be all she appeared when [he] first met her at the door . . ." (77). In this case, I use brackets to indicate changes I have made to fit the quotation to the grammatical structure of my sentence.

Part 3: Assignment

You are required to write an analytical essay, not an informal discussion of or response to literature. An analytical essay presents an argument about how and why an author does certain things in his or her work; it examines the work's thematic, conceptual, or rhetorical infrastructure (infrastructure means "the basic, underlying framework or features of a system"). Textual analysis is not limited to discovering "what the author intended"; often, the purpose of textual analysis is to explore the cultural, historical, and/or philosophical implications of the text's apparent or implicit design, the patterns of ideas, images, language, and/or themes in the text, and the gaps or breaks in those patterns. In this way, reading a text is a way to learn how to be a better reader of one's world, of the cultural forces that shape one's thinking, one's personality, even one's adopted role in life. Textual analysis can make one conscious of all those things that one sees and does unconsciously on a daily basis; it can help us defamiliarize and thereby see and think about our familiar customs and surroundings.

I expect you to write a formal analytical essay even if you have not done so before. If you have never written this kind of paper, and if you have no experience reading texts analytically, I recommend that you look at Mortimer J. Adler's and Charles Van Doren's *How to Read a Book*, an excellent book (and not as simplistic as its title suggests). If you are an experienced analytical reader, and if you would like to develop your skills by thinking about theoretical approaches to literary criticism, I recommend that you look at *Critical Terms for Literary Study*. Finally, if you would like to increase your critical vocabulary, develop your understanding of terms that I mention in class, familiarize yourself with literary genres and periods, and read introductions to various critical theories, look through M. H. Abrams's *A Glossary of Literary Terms* (especially the sixth edition). All of these books are listed in the Works Cited at the end of this guide, and all should be available at our library, or you could order your own copies through local bookstores.

Remember that textual analysis is a formal academic discipline and that every paper you write for me will test your mastery of its principles. Let me stress that point: the papers are tests. When you write, then, your task is to demonstrate your ability to present a persuasive analysis, as well as to present your analysis in a coherent and grammatically correct format.

If you are not sure that you know how to write the kind of paper I am requiring, please don't hesitate to ask for advice or help. I will be happy to help you with each stage of the writing process.

Part 4: The Introduction

Your introductory paragraph should have three stages (three stages but only one paragraph). In a longer essay (twenty pages or more), you would cover these same stages but in three or more paragraphs. The three stages are as follows:

1. In the first stage, you introduce your subject—the text itself. In a few (two to four) sentences, you should present the author and title of the work, along with a general overview of the work's plot, outstanding themes, or general achievement. The shorter the paper, the shorter this introductory passage should be; and in a very long essay (twenty-five to thirty pages), the first few pages might well be devoted to this introductory passage.

2. In the next stage, you present your topic—the interpretive issue to which your paper is devoted. In a sense, you need to show that there is cause for confusion and misunderstanding, or that there is a dimension of the work that is not clear unless one looks at it a certain way (for example, by viewing it within its historical context). You might establish the interpretive problem or issue in a number of ways:

    •   explain the problem or issue for the reader.

    •   open with a question which you develop in the opening paragraph.

    •   use a passage from the work to illustrate the problem or issue.

3. In the third stage, you present your thesis—your answer to the questions or issues you raise in stage 2. Your thesis should be explicit and specific. Consider carefully the following discussion of the thesis.

Do not begin your essay from the beginning of time. Postpone your comments about your personal feelings or response to the work, and postpone also your comments on the twentieth century when writing on literature from previous centuries. Usually, you can present material like this in your concluding paragraph, as you indicate the implications of the argument you have just presented. Get to the point elegantly, gracefully, directly, and quickly.

Part 5: The Thesis

An argument demonstrates the justice, value, and logical coherence of a *thesis*. Remember that a thesis is different from a subject or topic. The subject is the text you are analyzing. The topic is the interpretive issue you are trying to address. **The thesis is the stand you take on that issue.** A subject is what you are talking about; a topic is why you are talking about it; a thesis is what you are trying to say about that topic. A thesis is debatable; a topic is not, for a topic simply identifies—notes the existence of—grounds for debate or cause for confusion. A topic is something you can mention to a professor without feeling nervous; a thesis keeps you up at night.

This is not a thesis: "Melville uses symbolism in *Moby Dick*." What kind of symbolism? How does he use it? To what purpose? Will you examine all examples of symbolism *in the novel? Again, this is not a thesis: "Hawthorne examines history in* The Marble Faun." You might develop this observation into a thesis by establishing the specific issue and taking a clear stand. Consider, for example, this statement from a published essay:

> When Hawthorne says that those who object to the unresolved mysteries of *The Marble Faun*'s ending do "not know how to read a Romance," he means, as his work itself shows, that insofar as they expect definite answers to their questions or an unambiguous moral to the story, they do not know how to read history either. (Michael 150)

True, this is a *long* thesis; and, true, it makes the idea behind it sound more complicated than it actually is. Still, this scholar's purpose is clear, and one can anticipate what he will argue in the rest of the essay, and why.

- If you present your topic in the form of a question, your topic and thesis might look like this:

> What are we to make of Melville's emphasis on "The Whiteness of the Whale" in *Moby Dick*; or *The Whale*? Although it is tempting

to assert that this "whiteness" has nothing to do with the complex and contested racial landscape of the nineteenth-century United States, the novel offers significant evidence that race is indeed the issue to which all other concerns in this novel must be related.

- If you present your topic by quoting a sentence from the text, your topic and thesis might look like this:

In his appendix to *Narrative of the Life of Frederick Douglass, An American Slave*, Douglass seems to worry about the implications of his comments on religion throughout the body of this text. "I have," he notes, "in several instances, spoken in such a tone and manner, respecting religion, as may possibly lead those unacquainted with my religious views to suppose me an opponent of all religion." But as he explains his distinction between "the Christianity of this land" and "the Christianity of Christ," Douglass reapplies his concerns and suggests that the White Christian reader is actually the one who should worry about being considered an opponent of all religion.

Part 6: Structure

Academic writing is very basic and straightforward. It is designed to allow one to read subtle arguments quickly. Accordingly, the structure of your argument is very important. Each paragraph should present a unified block of thought, a clear and significant stage of your argument. You should therefore avoid paragraphs that are too long (in a short essay, page-long paragraphs are too long, often a sign of unfocused thinking) or too short. As a general rule, each paragraph should have at least five sentences. Paragraphs with fewer sentences often indicate undeveloped or unsubstantiated thought. Each paragraph should build on what you have done in the previous paragraph, and should prepare your reader for what you will argue in the next paragraph. If you can move your paragraphs around without disturbing the nature of your argument, then you have not paid sufficient attention to the structure of your argument or have simply repeated yourself in the course of your paper.

My term for the structure of an academic essay is the "intellectual matrix" of the essay. The "intellectual matrix" is what you get when you read only the thesis statement and the topic sentence of each of your paragraphs (normally the first sentence of the paragraph). Just as your thesis indicates clearly the argumentative purpose of your paper, so should the first sentence of each paragraph, the topic sentence, indicate the argumentative purpose of that paragraph. I should be able to read only these

210 • Section 4

sentences to determine the logical design of your argument. In other words, I should be able to summarize your argument from those sentences alone. Roughly one third of your grade will be based on the extent to which the "intellectual matrix" of your paper provides me with an accurate overview of your argument, and also on your ability to construct a systematic, unified argument that builds from one stage (one paragraph) to the next.

Part 7: Content

Remember that your assignment is textual, historical, and/or cultural analysis, not plot summary, and not simply general or subjective historical commentary. In textual analysis, your task is to show the connections between what the author says and how she or he says it—in other words, to identify and examine the implications of the author's strategies (style, themes, images, patterns of thought and of argument, etc.).

Remember that your reader has read and thought about the text to which your paper is devoted, and therefore does not need to be reminded of the plot. **Do not simply summarize the plot.**

Historical commentary is useful, usually even necessary (in small doses), but use it wisely, make sure you know what you are talking about, and do not allow it to distract you from your main task: informed analysis. Typically, the more general and abstract the historical context, the less useful it will be. Keep in mind that all people in a given time period did not think the same way, even if there are issues and ideas that did preoccupy many; be attentive, in other words, to conflicts, differences, and changes among groups within a period, and never claim that "nineteenth-century African Americans thought that . . ." Even more important, if you introduce historical commentary, you must take care that you provide some evidence for your historical claims and that you establish your historical context efficiently and succinctly. If you are using elements from an author's biography, for example, choose those elements that are relevant to your thesis and make sure that you establish why those elements are important for understanding the work.

Grades for papers based primarily on plot summary or on general historical commentary will begin somewhere in the area of a "C"—and they will go down from there.

You must present your argument carefully, methodically. In the early part of your paper, explain carefully the interpretive problem you intend to solve, and then proceed to solve it in stages. At each point of your paper, think about what your reader needs to know if he or she is to understand what is coming up in the next stage of your paper. At each stage, quote from your sources or from your primary text to show the basis for your interpretation. Show your reader that you are analyzing your topic or text and not just talking about it.

Focus is the key to success. You cannot hope to analyze an entire book, an entire century, or an entire social movement in a short paper. Therefore, you must isolate a representative portion of your topic. If you are writing about a literary text, for example, you might focus on a character, a scene, a rhetorical or ideological pattern, a pattern of allusions, or some other aspect of the author's techniques and strategies. Find something you can examine in detail and explain your interpretation carefully. Justify your choice at the beginning of your essay; at the end of your essay, indicate how your conclusions can enable readers to understand other aspects of the work.

Part 8: Research and Support—A Reminder

It is important to remember that you must support your claims, and that you must not make any claims that you are unable or unwilling to support. When you present an interpretation of a sentence or passage or episode in a text, you must explain carefully how the text supports that interpretation. If you make a point about history, then you must do the necessary historical research, and you must refer to that research in your essay (see me on how to do this if you have not done this before). If you say something about an author, then you must support that point with biographical research. If you say something about how critics have viewed a certain text, then you must support that with research. Avoid making claims about how readers respond to a certain text, for you cannot support such claims.

Part 9: Using Quotations

To present a persuasive argument, you must quote from the text you are analyzing, and you must explain carefully how the evidence you present leads to and supports your interpretation of the work. This is not to say that you should be blatant about this; that is, you shouldn't lead into a quotation by saying, "This interpretation is supported by the following quotation." Consider the following guidelines:

1. I should be convinced of the significance of the textual evidence (quotations from and allusions to the works) you present. That is, don't just quote. Prepare your reader for the textual evidence you will present; present that evidence briefly (avoid long quotations);

and then explicate, analyze, or otherwise explain the significance of that evidence. Never assume that a passage is self-explanatory.

2. Don't just present a quotation without introduction. I shouldn't suddenly encounter a quotation at the beginning of a new sentence, and you should never present a free-standing quotation (that is, a sentence that contains nothing but a quotation); always lead into the quotation in your own words, and then follow it with commentary.

3. Never end a paragraph with a quotation. Always follow with commentary, so that you conclude each of your paragraphs with your own words.

4. Avoid long quotations. Whenever possible, integrate significant phrases from the text in your own sentences as you present and explain your interpretation.

5. Whenever you use a significant word or phrase from the text, use quotation marks to indicate that you are in fact using someone else's words.

The following is taken from one of my essays, "From Mysteries to Histories: Cultural Pedagogy in Frances E. W. Harper's *Iola Leroy*." I present this so that you can have a model for using quotations, but I do not expect you to simply imitate my style. Indeed, I wish you the good fortune of avoiding my overly complex style. Still, I hope you will find it useful to examine (and, perhaps, question) my use of textual evidence.

From the Essay

Harper establishes the terms of this argument, and begins the novel, by confronting her white readers with their inability to interpret culturally-familiar discourse. In the first pages of the first chapter, Harper draws readers into a "shadow" culture—that of the slaves—and introduces her readers to the discursive network of that culture, the "mystery of market speech." Her depiction of slaves talking enthusiastically about "splendid" fish, and about butter "just as fresh, as fresh can be" (7-8) invokes images of the stereotypical Black characters who inhabited the pages of white supremacist fiction gaining popularity at the time. On the novel's second page, though, the narrator wonders at this "unusual interest manifested by these men in the state of the produce market," and raises the question that many readers might well have forgotten to ask: "What did it mean?" (8). The answer is that, during the war, "when the bondman was turning his eyes to the American flag," "some of the shrewder slaves . . . invented a phraseology to convey in the most unsuspected manner news to each other from the battle-field" (8-9). The "mystery of market speech" is thus solved by learning this phraseology, this cultural discourse that appropriates authorized, and in that sense, legal language for illegal but moral ends.

The primary point here is not that this particular mystery is now clear, nor is it merely that the slaves had to formulate their own language to circumvent the will of the dominant race; rather, the point lies in the discursive nature of the mystery itself, the extent to which one's ability to understand is controlled by one's cultural training. As one reads, one encounters other such mysteries, each of which reveals the cognitive and moral limitations inherent in and enforced by the dominant cultural system. Consider, for example, Dr. Gresham, whom the reader first meets in a field hospital, and who is clearly attracted to Iola Leroy, whom he believes to be a white lady generously lowering herself to serve the needs of the Northern soldiers. Initially, Dr. Gresham cannot understand how Iola can bring herself to kiss a black patient; and as he explains this to Col. Robinson, the reader discovers the terms of his confusion:

> I cannot understand how a Southern lady, whose education and manners stamp her as a woman of fine culture and good breeding, could consent to occupy the position she so faithfully holds. It is a mystery I cannot solve. (57)

This description is essentially a circular equation of cultural identity. If one is a Southern lady, then one must have the advantages of education and good breeding which provide the manners and fine culture that are, by definition, the qualities of a Southern lady. The perfect circle of definition represents the cognitive closure that is the raison d'etre of any culture system. When this closure leads to culturally exotic behavior, those within the cultural circle are faced with a mystery they cannot solve. When Col. Robinson provides the essential information, that "Miss Leroy was a slave," Dr. Gresham can relocate her in the cultural formula, and he says revealingly, "What you tell me changes the whole complexion of affairs" (58). Dr. Gresham, in other words, is able to relocate Iola according to existing cultural categories and stereotypes.

Note on using quotations: In the example from my own writing, note how the material from the work is integrated with my own words, and how I combine both block quotation and in-text quotation to incorporate the evidence into the prose. The idea is to make sure that yours is the dominant voice in your writing, that you prepare your reader for the quotations, and that your essay is as smooth as possible. Try these techniques in your own work.

Part 10: A Sample Works Cited Page (MLA format)

Note: Different academic disciplines (Literature, History, etc.) require different approaches to documentation; most do not use the MLA format. Always check your syllabus, or check with your professor, to determine what form you should use.

Works Cited

Abrams, M. H. *A Glossary of Literary Terms*. 6th ed. Fort Worth: Harcourt Brace, 1993.

Adler, Mortimer J., and Charles Van Doren. *How to Read a Book*. Revised and Updated Edition. A Touchstone Book. New York: Simon & Schuster, 1972.

Ernest, John. "From Mysteries to Histories: Cultural Pedagogy in Frances E. W. Harper's Iola Leroy." *American Literature* 64 (1992): 497-518.

Gibaldi, Joseph, and Walter S. Achtert. *MLA Handbook for Writers of Research Papers*. Third Edition. New York: The Modern Language Association of America, 1988.

Lentricchia, Frank, and Thomas McLaughlin, eds. *Critical Terms for Literary Study*. Chicago: Univ. of Chicago Press, 1990.

Michel, John. "History and Romance, Sympathy and Uncertainty: The Moral of the Stones in Hawthorne's Marble Faun." *PMLA* 103 (1988): 150-161.

How to Write Clearly, Concisely, and Effectively

Dr. John Burger

Zoology

Effective writing is hard work. If you wish to write clearly and effectively, as well as hold the reader's interest, you can produce written communication that you will be proud to call your own. The following information and tips will help you communicate scientific and technical topics effectively and avoid terminology, phrases, and sentence structure that can be confusing to the reader. If followed conscientiously, they will improve your writing skills and ability to communicate your ideas and those of others to the reader. This is by no means a comprehensive guide, but is based largely on writing encountered in this class's past writing assignments, discussions at the University of Writing Center, and with Margaret Moore and Ann Stork, whose comments and suggestions are gratefully acknowledged.

First Things First:
The Stages in Preparing a Writing Assignment.

Preparing a good written assignment can be divided into six stages, beginning with planning, and ending with sentence-level editing/ proofreading.

1. **Freewriting/Brainstorming.** This is the stage when you write about the main ideas you wish to present. Consider whether you will write from an outline, directly from literature sources or other information, or from notes on your information sources. Use what works best for you. Get all your thoughts and ideas down on paper.

2. **Discuss ideas with peers.** During this stage, get comments from peers or anybody else that you think can comment on the ideas

you will present. This will be very helpful in identifying the main themes of the paper and clarifying thoughts and ideas, or even expressing them in a different way or in a different order.

3. **Compose the first draft.** For this stage, you do only *one* thing: *write, write, write.* Don't worry about how it sounds or if the organization is good or everything is spelled correctly, *just write!* Use your "writing brain" and keep your "revising/editing brain" turned off. Get it all down on paper. Don't try to edit while you write. It inhibits the creative process. Have others read and comment on your rough draft or submit it to your instructor.

4. **Revise for clear statement and flow of ideas.** Now, turn on your "revising brain." This is the "global" process of revision. You examine the paper as a whole, not its individual parts. Is the organization clear? Is your focus appropriate to the topic area? Have you included as many concepts as are required to adequately cover the assigned topic? How thorough is your presentation? Is more information needed to cover the topic well?

5. **Paragraph-level organization and editing.** During this stage, examine each entire paragraph carefully. Does each paragraph deal with one idea and one idea only? If more than one idea is presented in a paragraph, it should be divided into two paragraphs. Does the first sentence of the paragraph introduce the idea clearly? Does the last sentence of the paragraph provide a "lead in" for the next paragraph? Does paragraph organization flow smoothly? Examine paragraph level *only*.

6. **Sentence-level editing and proofreading.** This is absolutely the last stage in the writing process. Now, you turn on your "editing brain" and look at sentence structure for the following "magic words": Positive, Precise and Concise. Here, you will check for misspelling, mixed use of singular and plural nouns and verbs, position of the "Agent of Action" (see below) in the sentence, use of unnecessary or imprecise words and phrases, inappropriate use of the passive voice, use of "conversational" language, and punctuation. You will maximize "readability" and "clarity."

The following suggestions will assist you in this last process. Most examples are taken from actual papers written by students in ZOOL 690.

Proofreading

You *must* proofread your writing carefully to avoid careless or inadvertent mistakes in spelling, grammar and style. Careful proofreading will ensure that your work is well-written and clear. It also indicates that you care about what you write. Here are two strategies I use to proofread the papers I write:

1. Cover your texts with a blank card or sheet of opaque paper and read one line at a time. Do not move to the next line until you have read *every* word of the previous line and understand its meaning. Check for words or phrases that are not clear and correct them, or mark them for subsequent correction. Eyes have a tendency to skip over words, or even sentences, especially when you have read the material before. This will prevent skipping over words until the line has been read completely. This is "fine tuning." Use a *printed* hard copy.

2. Read the text out loud or have a friend or roommate read it to you out loud. You will be amazed how different written material can sound when read aloud. It also helps you catch words or phrases that do not make sense or seem inappropriate.

Suggestions for concise writing

*   Eliminate the word "the" when it is not necessary to the meaning of the sentence. It is used far more often than necessary. Example: "In the experience the body size was manipulated . . ." "In the experiment body size was manipulated . . ." [Note: This is also a terrible example because (a) it is in the passive voice (see below), and (b) the sentence begins with a preposition (in). You should avoid both!]

*   Avoid use of words and phrases that do not contribute to the meaning of sentences. This distracts the reader from the points you are making. This is called "wordiness."

*   Notice how many of the following examples are used commonly in conversational speech or use the passive voice.

Examples of wordiness and how to avoid it.

Wordy	Concise
a	
a total of	unnecessary—give number
a lot of	unnecessary—give number
advancements	advances
allowed for	allowed
allows for this	allows
almost all	most (imprecise!!!)
along side [of]	with
an effort is made here to	I attempt to
as determined by	determined by
as it stands now	present
as of now	now
as seen in	in
as to how	how
at that moment	then
b	
backed up	supported
broken down into/by	subdivided into/by
brought about	caused
brought forward	presented
c	
called into question	questioned/disputed
came about	occurred
came into being	originated
came to be	originated
came up with	proposed
can be taken to be	can be
caused there to be	resulted in
d	
divided up	divided
done away with	eliminated
due to the fact that	because

f

falls near the realm of	is related, close to, near
first off	first

g

gave support for	supported
goes in direct conflict with	conflicts with
goes on to	then
grounded on	based on

h

had its foundation in	originated
have come to be used	are used
have to do with	deal with, pertain to
hold that a belief	believes
how it is that	how can

i

in a similar manner	similar, similarly
in addition to this	also, additionally, etc.
in an attempt to	attempted to, attempts to
in comparison to	compared to (or with)
in hopes that	hoping
in no way	not
in order to figure out	to explain
in order to/for	to, for
in regard[s] to	concerning, regarding
in respect to	regarding
in support of	to support
in terms of	in
in the end	finally
in this day and age	at present
is lacking in	lacks
is objected to	is questioned, disputed
it is also believed	_____ believes
it was thought by some	some thought (but who is "some"?)
it was thought by many	many thought (how many?)

k

keep in mind	remember

l

later on	later
lean more toward	favor
lends support to	supports
liked to believe	believed
looked upon	considered

m

make the conclusion that	conclude
more and more	increasingly

n

nonexistence/nonexistent	absent

o

oftentimes	often
on an individual basis	individually
on behalf of	by, for
on the basis of	based on, by
on the order of	about, approximately

p

point to	use
pretty much	nearly
put across	explain
put down	criticized

r

read into	interpret

s

scrutinization	scrutiny
so long as	if
solid evidence	convincing evidence
somewhere on the order of	about, approximately
stick around	persist
stretches out	extends
sums up	summarizes
survivability	survival

t

take into consideration	consider
that embodies the belief that	states
that looked at	examined
the inclusion of	include
the things that he watched for	he observed
the ways in which	how
they concluded the study by capturing	they captured
through Stephen Jay Gould, we are reminded	Stephen Jay Gould reminds us
to back the conclusion up	support the conclusion
to further the advancement of	to advance
to look more closely at	examine [closely]
to try and find	try to find
toss aside	reject

u

up until	until
usage	use
utilized/utilization	use, used

w

was born out of	originated
was in opposition to	opposed
was lacking in	lacked
whether or not	if
why it is that	why do
with an association to	associated with
with the aim of	to
within	in

Do Not Use the Following Wordy/Meaningless Words/Phrases:

"in other words"
"overall"
"for the most part"
"along the same lines"
"as previously stated"

"on the other hand"
"it is quickly noted"
"as you can tell"
"in a way"
"countless"

"in the process of"	"based on this"
"as mentioned earlier"	"upward of"
"it was found that"	"be able to be"
"it can be seen that"	"in the way of"
"lastly"	"at the age of"

These are called "running jumps" and usually obscure the meaning of sentences.

Suggestions for Precise Writing

Precise writing helps the reader understand your written work and minimizes confusion. It also allows the reader to read your entire work without pausing to puzzle out what you mean. The following examples deal with precision.

- Do not use "some" to refer to specific groups of individuals—it is too vague—identify the "some" more specifically. Same applies to "many," unless you specify who the "many" are.
- Beware when using the word "this." Its meaning can be vague—be sure you clearly indicate what "this" is and to what it refers.
- Beware of starting sentences with "in" (or other prepositions). It usually means your main idea is buried somewhere in the middle of the sentence. It can indicate use of the passive voice. Do not end sentences with prepositions, if possible (in, of, about). Example: "In *Darwin on Trial*, Johnson discusses this." "Johnson discusses this in *Darwin on Trial*." *Do not* begin sentences with a phrase whose first word is "By" or whose first word is an "ing" word. It is a sure sign that the main idea/subject (agent of action) is buried deep in the sentence's interior and will make the sentence more difficult to read and understand.
- Avoid using "conversational English" and "slang" whenever possible (see also examples under concise writing). It usually makes what you are trying to express more difficult to understand. What is commonly used and acceptable in conversation often is not appropriate in written communication or has a different meaning. For example, "on the other hand" means what? What and whose hand do you mean, left or right? How many hands are there? Another excellent example is "incredible." It is commonly used in conversation to mean "great" or "super" or "especially good" or "wonderful." But the written word actually means "not believable"

or "not to be believed." If you are not "credible," you are not to be believed, so you are incredible!

- Always be *careful* about using the words "they," "it," "many," "some." Be sure to clearly link these words to the agents they represent, or better, avoid them when possible!

Examples of Imprecision and How to Fix Them

Imprecise/Vague	Clear
in depth	detailed
upon	on
as to	about
a lack of	no, little, etc.
realize	understand
as opposed to	rather than, instead of, in contrast to
made up of	composed of
breaks down, broken down by	divides, subdivides, subdivided by
deal with	pertain to
pushed	supported
to back up the conclusion	support
as	because
ran into	encountered
somewhere on the order of	about, approximately

Do Not Use These Imprecise Terms or Phrases:

fell into	
big, bigger	
a vast number of	
in	*Not* at beginning of sentence
which vs. that	Don't use "which" when you mean "that." When in doubt, "that" is usually preferable.

Word Confusion

Be careful in your use of words. For example, don't use "affect" when you mean "effect," or "effect" when you mean "affect." Affect refers to an action (remember A for action!!) and is a verb. Effect can be either a noun or a verb. Another example: do not use "data is." Data is plural; datum is singular. Its or it's. Its implies possession; it's is a contraction for "it is."

Passive Voice Disease

Don't use the passive voice excessively. Better not to use it at all, or only sparingly. Passive voice sentences tend to have "weak" verbs. Simple, declarative sentences are usually MUCH clearer and easier to read and understand. Examples of "passive voice disease": "It was believed by many that . . ." "It was thought by many that . . ." Use instead: "many believe", "many thought." [Note: but watch out for "many" unless you specify what many you mean.]

The Agent of Action

One way to ensure that you will write clear, strong sentences that are easy to read and understand is to identify the "agent of action" (AOA) in each sentence and place it as close to the beginning of the sentence as possible. Example: "Looking at one very specific aspect of the Nazi movement, in this case the burning of books, which went along with the suppression of ideas and positive progress, anyone today would say this was a horrible occurrence." The AOA here is "anyone" (in boldface), but you have to read most of the sentence before you reach it. Here is a revised sentence with the AOA near the beginning: "Today, anyone who examined particular events during the Nazi era, such as book burning and suppression of ideas, would consider it horrible." The first sentence has thirty-seven words. The revised version has twenty-two words, but the meaning of the sentence has not changed, and is clearer and easier to read.

Other Issues

- Beware of the "dangling" phrase! Example: "In order to obtain samples from Great Bay, a van was taken by the students." A less awkward and verbose way to express this is: "The students drove a van to Great Bay to collect samples." [not an example from the writing exercises]. More about beginning and ending sentences with prepositions below. Be certain the sentence says what you want it to say. The following examples clearly do NOT say what the author intended:
  1. "Originally created as a model bill for California creationists, the Act made its way through fundamentalist channels and ended up in Arkansas, authored by Paul Ellwanger." Here, the AOA ("the Act") is in the middle of the sentence, and I

don't think Paul Ellwanger authored Arkansas, but that is what the sentence says!

2. "The factors come together to make an interesting story about the ever-changing world of 14 finches on a group of islands that evolved from one ancestor." I doubt that the islands evolved from one ancestor, but that is what the sentence says!

3. "Magazines depicted Darwin having a monkey-shaped body sitting in a tree with a long tail." I don't think the tree really had a long tail, but that is what the sentence says!

4. "Hybridization supports the common ancestor theory by showing that different species are so similar in structure and function that they can interbreed and produce offspring even though sterile." Hard to see how a sterile organism could interbreed and produce offspring, but that is what the sentence says!

5. "Fossil anthropologists claim, 'Lucy shows nothing about human evolution.'" I don't think the writer really mean that anthropologists were fossils, but that is what the sentence says!

6. "Through overuse and misuse bacterial microbes have evolved and have become resistant to many of the antibiotics that once were able to kill them." Hard to figure out how bacterial microbes are misused and overused and I am not certain how bacterial microbes that were killed by antibiotics came back to life again and became resistant, but that is what the sentence says!

7. "A mutation in a biology text says: 'A rare change in the DNA of genes that ultimately creates genetic diversity . . .'" I don't think the writer really meant to say that it was a mutant biology text, but that is what the sentence says!

8. "By dating fossils in sedimentary rock, geologists can form a fossilized time scale." The sentence begins with "By," the AOA is buried in the middle of the sentence, and I don't think time scales are fossilized, but that is what the sentence says!

    •   Be careful with punctuation, especially commas (Random Comma Disease). There were many examples of commas where they were not appropriate and no commas where they were required. Example: "In the experiment body size was manipulated" should be: "in the experiment, body size was manipulated" BUT this is passive voice and the sentence begins with "in"; instead, use: "_____ manipulated body size in the experiment." The University Writing Center can help you master punctuation. A good way to check on punctuation is to read the sentences aloud. You will notice natural breaks in sentence cadence. This often is a hint where commas should (or should not) be.

A cat has claws at the end of its paws.

A comma's a pause at the end of a clause.

• You might be tempted to say "Big Deal!" But bungled punctuation can completely change the meaning of a statement. Consider the two following examples from Lynne Truss's book *Eats, Shoots & Leaves*, whose title is taken from a bungled translation of a Chinese wildlife manual about giant pandas. The following two passages have exactly the same words in the same order, but opposite meanings due to differences in punctuation:

A woman, without her man, is nothing.

A woman: without her, man is nothing.

Dear Jack,
I want a man who knows what love is all about. You are generous, kind, thoughtful. People who are not like you admit to being useless and inferior. You have ruined me for other men. I yearn for you. I have no feelings whatsoever when we're apart. I can be happy forever—will you let me be yours?

Jill

Dear Jack,
I want a man who knows what love is. All about you are generous, kind, thoughtful people, who are not like you. Admit to being

useless and inferior. You have ruined me. For other men I yearn! For you I have no feelings whatsoever. When we're apart I can be happy forever. Will you let me be?

Yours, Jill

- Do not mix singular and plural nouns and verbs in the same sentence. Example: "For extremist they do not need any scientific evidence . . ."
- The "I" word. Until recently, personal pronouns were considered to be "no-nos" in scientific writing. No more!! It costs money to print journals, and editors encourage economy. If you did or thought or said or believe, say "I did", "I said", "I thought", "I think", "I believe(d)."

Avoid the Following:

lastly	last
and so on	*do not use*
firstly, secondly	first, second
Because of this	*do not* begin a sentence this way
It is believed	Indicative of "passive voice disease"

The Personal Touch

Does scientific or technical writing have to be (1) impersonal, (2) dry, (3) "objective" (whatever that is), (4) boring, (5) dull, (6) technical, (7) filled with specialized jargon? It certainly can be, but does not have to be. If you think so, why do Stephen Jay Gould, Edward O. Wilson, and Stephen Hawking make so much money writing books? Easy. Lots of people buy these books. Why? Because they are interesting and personal. These (and other) authors put the personal in their writing, especially for a general audience. You should do likewise when you write about scientific or technical topics. I guarantee that your writing will be far more interesting to read. This does not mean your writing should be imprecise or "colloquial"—but engage the reader!! You'll be glad you did. And so will the reader!!